Fitface

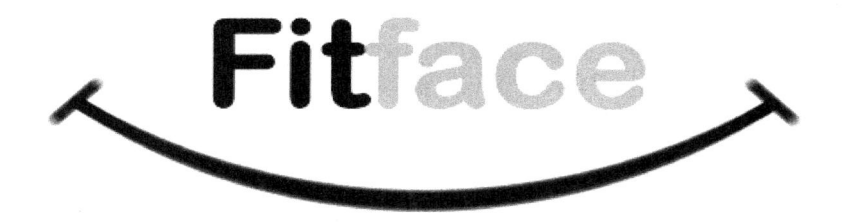

Fitface Facial Exercises

The book of face and neck exercises

CHARLOTTE HAMILTON

First Copyright © 2008 Charlotte Hamilton
Copyright © 2010, 2012 Text and photographs

Fitface - Volume 3
Fitface Facial Exercises
The book of face and neck exercises

First published 2012
ISBN-13: 978-1475022841
ISBN-10: 1475022840

All rights reserved
No part of this publication may be reproduced or transmitted in any form or by any means, electronic or mechanical, including photocopy, recording or any information storage and retrieval system, without written permission from the author and/or publisher.

For bulk order purchases or for other information please visit

Fitface Website http://www.fitfacetoning.com
Fitface email fitfacetoning@aol.com
Fitface Blog http://blog.fitfacetoning.com
Fitface Twitter https://twitter.com/#!/Fitfacetoning
Facebook Fitface Toning http://www.facebook.com/fitface.toning

YouTube videos
http://www.youtube.com/user/Fitfacetoning?feature=mhee
FITFACE 5pm News May 2010
http://www.youtube.com/watch?v=IZ32IgoC_xQ&context=C4de9eb8ADv
jVQa1PpcFOAbvj0Q1NWJwCysi4u0LA2ZpyfDhCfaK0=
FITFACE Hands free toning fun
http://www.youtube.com/watch?v=xVCgx9XWg0E&context=C450a120A
DvjVQa1PpcFOAbvj0Q1NWJw5WKJZIVbAWZ7UUm33jNaQ=
Fitface Toning Home Study Course
http://www.youtube.com/watch?v=IYDVzEf_KrA
Fitface facial exercises seminar
http://www.youtube.com/watch?v=_NS-JEWJSVk
Me, being me at Christmas 2011
http://www.youtube.com/watch?v=CK4Fy8Qipdg&context=C459d609AD
vjVQa1PpcFOAbvj0Q1NWJ0yMuxEWRYLWaLj0KJUY1wY=

Published typeset, printed and bound in the United States

By the same author

Charlotte Hamilton

Fitface: Hands Free Facial Toning Exercises

Digital
http://www.amazon.com/Fitface-ebook/dp/B0049H9538
Paperback
http://www.amazon.com/Fitface-Hands-Facial-Toning-Exercises/dp/1453777830

Fitface Foundations
Exercises only - extracted from
Fitface: Hands Free Facial Toning Exercises

Digital
http://www.amazon.com/Fitface-Foundations-ebook/dp/B005LB7XZ8
Paperback
http://www.amazon.com/Fitface-Foundations-Exercises-Charlotte-Hamilton/dp/1463665687

Out of print
Fitface: The natural facelift

Under the pseudonym Colette Sinclair
MAN HUNT

First published 1989
Sidgwick and Jackson - Pan Macmillan Press

This book is a work of non-fiction and a true story.

To respect the sensibilities of some people and the professional careers of others, I have elected to purposefully withhold some names throughout the book.

Liability Waiver

Fitface Toning Inc accepts no responsibility or liability for any injury, loss or damage to any party undertaking or performing the facial exercises, stretches or procedures set out within this book and all parties undertake and perform such exercises, movements, stretches and procedures entirely at their own risk.

The reader further acknowledges, agrees and understands that the information here within is for reference and education only and not in any way intended to be a substitute for a physician's advice, diagnosis or treatment.

About the Author

Born and raised in England. Charlotte immigrated to California USA in her twenties. There she witnessed firsthand the butchery of a major facelift to her former partner and vowed never to have a facelift. Following the breakup of her marriage she returned to England to raise her new baby daughter. Eighteen years later, her daughter suffered a horrendous near fatal accident in which she sustained major facial trauma with 21 fractures to her face. She survived, graduated from a British University with an honours' degree and now lives in Australia.

Charlotte returned briefly to live in Florida USA, but following a fall sustained by her elderly mother she returned to live in the South of England where she still resides.

Charlotte loves to hear from her readers and will endeavour to answer every single e-mail. She invites you to visit her website at www.Fitfacetoning.com

Fitface

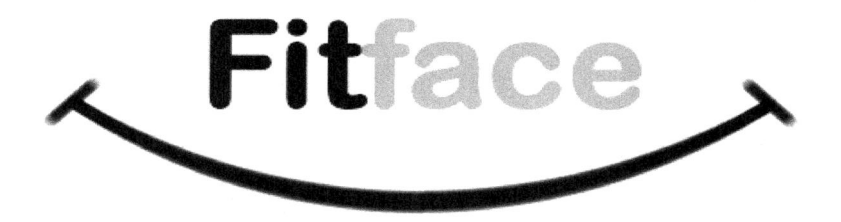

Fitface Facial Exercises

The book of face and neck exercises

Nature's beauty spa

Fitface Contents

Part 1 0
Information you need to know

Chapter 1 2
Fitface's mission is to encourage you to explore the benefits of facial exercise

Fitface's Primary Mission 2
Fitface's Secondary Mission 8
Ultimate Fitface Mission 11
The Fitface Vision 12
The History of Fitface 12
Hands free development 14
The book on face and neck exercises 19
Chinese eye exercises 25
Photos of me growing up 30
Fitface techniques and methods are simple 37
We all age but Fitface puts health before beauty 37
Fitface is nature's beauty spa 37
Images 39
Plastic Surgery: Keeping Celebrities Looking Old and Stupid 47

Chapter 2 50
How and why Fitface will make you look radiant

Why we age 50
How to prevent premature aging 50
How to glow with healthy good looks 50
Natural facial aging phenomena 52
Communication 52
Visible signs of facial aging 55
How to have a healthy glowing skin 57
Face exercise for your five sense organs 65
Why Facial Exercises Are Good For You 66
Why do facial exercises? 67
Exercise increases collagen 70
What can Fitface do for you? 70
Top 10 reasons to do "hands free" facial exercises 72
Why does exercise stop at the neck? 72

Chapter 3 86
What wrinkles are and how to erase them

Muscles of Facial Expression 86
Anatomically 87
An overview of wrinkle formation and how to erase them ... 88
There are three forms of wrinkles 90
Static wrinkles 91
Dynamic wrinkles 91
Wrinkle folds 92
How the body works 92
How muscles grow 92
How muscles move 95
Muscles learn 101

The skin 102
Epidermis 103
Dermis 106
The Subcutis (Subcutaneous fatty tissue) 107
Collagen 108
Elastin 112

Chapter 4 114
The alternatives to Fitface

Facial exercise methods 117
Topical treatments 118
Creams 118
Over the counter creams 118
Skin lipid replacement products 126
Are very expensive skin creams worth the price? 126
Non invasive treatments 127
Gadgets & treatments 127
Invasive procedures 135
The slippery slope of dependency leading to addiction 135
Flab jab by syringe 137
Injectables by needle 137
What are the side effects of BOTOX®? 138
Tissue fillers 141
Extremely invasive procedures 143
Surgically implants 143
Cosmetic surgery 143
My opinion on cosmetic facial surgery 145
The psychological effects of cosmetic surgery 146
The future for the cosmetics industry 146

Part 2 150

10-minute face exercise routines

Chapter 5 152

Exercise routines

6 for each part of your face
5 for each week day

The Fitface Toning Guidelines	153
WEEKLY ROUTINE	156
DAILY ROUTINE	158
THE WARM UP	160
THE EXERCISES	161
THE COOL DOWN	163

The Exercises

Fitface - 50 "hands free" face and neck exercises

Skin care	168
Warm Up Exercises 1 - 16	168
Exercises Whole face 1-6	200
Exercises Mouth (Lower face) 1-6	212
Exercises Eyes 1-6	224
Exercises Mouth (Upper face) 1-6	236
Exercises Neck 1-6	248
Cool Down 1 - 4	258

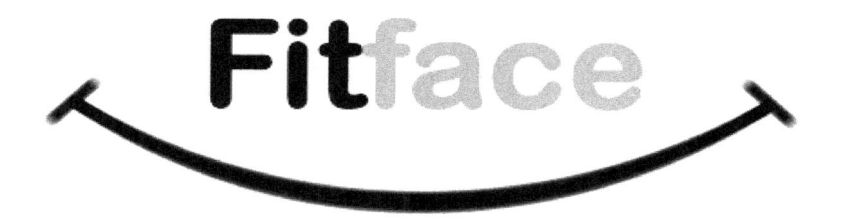

Fitface Facial Exercises

Information you need to know

Part 1

Chapter 1

Fitface - Nature's beauty spa

Fitface's missions

Fitface development and history
Fitface's techniques
Celebrity images

I want to raise awareness of the benefits of "hands-free" facial toning and to empower my readers with knowledge, on how and why Fitface face and neck exercises encourage glowing skin, prevent wrinkles and can remove fine lines. Whereas creams are disappointing and the alternatives of needles or knives exacerbate wrinkles in the long-term and promote a never ending expensive, painful and risky cycle of dependency. Fitface is safe, affordable, and natural. Fitface feels good - try it - what have you got to lose? Only dull skin and premature signs of aging!

Fitface's primary mission

To show women and men that there is a natural long lasting way to have glowing skin and hair, postpone wrinkles or folds and erase lines. The informed choice is Fitface.
The face is covered with a connected system of muscles and collagen-rich connective tissue responsible for smiling, frowning and other facial expressions. Facial exercises are essential for a youthful glowing healthy-looking face regardless of age. The exercise movements boast circulation which brings extra oxygen and nutrients to your face and head to improve your skin and hair.

Face exercise builds collagen and muscle fibres that cover your whole face gives your face fullness, structure, tone and definition. Facial exercises are like going to the spa for your face.

The King of Fitness – Jack LaLanne was passionate about facial exercise and almost all of his exercises were performed "hands free" like mine in Fitface; see many of his on YouTube where there are over 30 facial workouts. He remained fit and healthy all his life until he died at the age of 96 and still looked good for his age. So he must have been doing something right!
http://en.wikipedia.org/wiki/Jack_LaLanne

To reason that exercise should not stop at the neck.
Everyone agrees that body exercises are "good" for you. Then surely it follows that face exercises are "good" for you as well?! Why not invigorate and tone your face with Fitface? Moreover, should it not be especially important since all the sense organs of touch, sight, sound taste and smell are located in our head as well as the brain? Would they not benefit from increased exercise which we all understand makes for strong healthy tissues?

In China it is mandatory for school children to do facial exercises twice daily for eyesight alone! Can almost one and half billion people in China be wrong? Exercise strengthens muscle fibres.

To demonstrate that ONLY facial exercises can stimulate natural growth of muscle tissues and collagen in the face.
Collagen molecules cannot penetrate the outer layers of the skin in a face cream, and therefore, the harvested bovine (cattle) collagen replacements are **temporarily placed** under the skin by an injection, within a few months they disperse. However, with exercise, collagen is naturally produced there **permanently**. BOTOX® only relaxes those muscles that it is injected into, whereas facial exercises naturally relaxes all the facial muscles – to give you tone plus the benefit of a glowing healthy skin too. Face exercises have the same effect on your face as body exercises do on your body. Furthermore, they produce collagen but not elastin because it **cannot** be produced by the normal human body past puberty; the **only artificial** way to stimulate elastin growth is Growth Hormone, which is dangerous and unnatural.

To assist men and women in making a logical decision about how to prevent premature natural facial aging.
Face exercises should naturally be the preferred option as there are no unknown negative side effects in the short or long-term. An alternative, such as the neurotoxin BOTOX® has only been FDA approved since 2002.But, just 7 years later, in 2009 Allergen, (the manufacturer) was ordered by the F.D.A. to put the strongest **"Black Box"** warning on the product. In effect, warning that amongst other side effects was death. The long-term effects are as yet unknown. There is conclusive evident that BOTOX® which is a neurotoxin can migrate/travel to the brain and other parts of the body. Worse there is a new physiological addiction called **'Wrinklerexia'** when some BOTOX® devotees become so obsessed with their wrinkle-free image that they start seeing lines where there are none and binge on BOTOX® to obtain a freeze-frame face.
FDA Slaps Black Box Warning on Botox, Other Anti-wrinkle Drugs
http://cherryhill.injuryboard.com/fda-and-prescription-drugs/fda-slaps-black-box-warning-on-botox-other-antiwrinkle-drugs.aspx?googleid=262208

To stop women getting on the slippery slope of dependency or addiction on needles that inevitably leads to knives.
The alternatives to face exercises are either ineffectual or risky and expensive; short term "quick fixes" that in the long-term cause more harm than good. A quick, short-term fix leads to a merry-go-round of ever more frequent, diminishing result, because the skin has been subjected to unnatural damage by the plumping out of the skin. Eventually, needles lead to the knives, which often lead to implants, which ultimately result in a freakish look that leads to more operations to try to correct the problem! Learn from others with the addiction.

This is just one comment I found from an acutely distressed Botox user who complained that she was not told in her consultation that having Botox would create the problem of incurring more wrinkles.

"To be honest this makes me a little upset. // you'd think that sales of this stuff would drop significantly if people knew this information more widely. you make it sound really simple like, well just get more product! oh great, so i have to keep spending $1500 a year

to keep fixing damage i got from spending $400?? That sounds like something a drug dealer would say. // i appreciate this stuff works fine for lots of people but it can't just be acceptable to say "well you might get a bunch of new wrinkles that look worse than the old ones, but i sure wont tell you that anywhere before you do it, but hey, give me some more money and i'll fix you up. and also, give you more wrinkles so you'll be stuck doing it again. yay for me!" that just sounds awful. will these effects go away completely on their own, or will they not? // if they will not, that needs to be made clearly known before people do this procedure. this was - never- listed in anything i read or saw about potential side effects. not cool."

To help all women and men understand how and why the faces ages and how to stay looking and acting younger longer naturally.
Whilst we all age, there are many things; we can do to slow the process one of the most important of which is body and facial exercising. Take your face to nature's beauty spa, Fitface.

To teach both men and women Fitface face exercises and explain the differences between Fitface "hand's free" facial toning and the other facial exercise routines available.
Fitface is "Hands-free", which means that there is no danger of undue or unnecessary pressure on the face and therefore no possibility of any over stretching of the delicate facial skin or internal damage to the elastin.

To encourage both men and women to start performing Fitface facial exercise when the first signs of aging appear; possibly in their late twenties or early thirties begin to build strong connections/neurological pathways in the brain.
Exercise, be it, the body or the face, are best started sooner rather than later. They are good habits than can last a lifetime. What goes in today will come out tomorrow, or later in life. Good habits become routine, a way of life – like brushing your teeth. Your face needs a natural spa break with Fitface.

To assure older women that they too can see positive results from doing facial exercises.
No matter how ever old you are it is never too late to start the facial exercises, their muscles will respond - be it slower. Not only

will it improve your facial tone, but mentally it will be a positive step in the right direction.

To expose the outdated old-fashioned notions and expel the myth that facial exercise causes wrinkle when as it is proven that Botox does!
The cosmetic surgery industry is a multibillion dollar that has tried to deflect attention from the benefits of facial exercise. Many cosmetic surgery clinics have multiple offices and huge turnover targets to achieve. Doctors are unlikely to turn away business at the "free" consultation and tell you to go home and exercise!

Hassan Galadari, MD 10 Nov 2010
"Further reading of the article explains how these wrinkles develop. When muscles that are injected become relaxed, a person who is new to Botox starts using other muscles for expressions he's used to make. This recruitment of other muscles causes more wrinkles. The most common area that gets affected by this is the bunny lines on the nose when the crow's feet are injected. It's easily remedied with a tad bit of material in the newly recruited muscle."
http://www.realself.com/forum/botox-give-wrinkles
So more addiction to jabs! Crazy – has the whole world gone mad or is it just me?

To explain why there is a conflict between cosmetic surgeons/dermatologists/the media and facial exercise.
Money is the real conflict. Cosmeceutical and pharmaceutical companies are enormously influential and have inexhaustible pockets full of huge funds to launch drugs and products on to the market be it via a doctor's office or media advertising. The TV/Radio/newspapers cannot (like everyone else) afford to bite the hand that feeds them or they would be out of business.

To help people to love themselves as they are and enhance what nature gave them with exercise rather than follow without questions pharmaceutical falsehoods.
Yes, Fitface is fantastic for you, both mentally and physically; the face does need exercise, just like the body, perhaps even more so. When you start Fitface you will be taking responsibility for who you are and how you look, it is a natural spa in a book. It will not make you look completely different, which should be positive!

Embrace who you are as an individual, stop to learn, to love the way you look, as the unique wonderful individual you are.

To ask the public to find out information independently and to think logically for themselves about facial aging and the money spent on over the counter face creams.
Regrettably, in today's world we cannot take information "at face value." Be it a leaflet through the door telling you that "you won" and must immediately claim your prize to a product saying it can stimulate elastin – **NO, it cannot! Elastin** stops reproducing at puberty. Furthermore Collagen molecules cannot independently get through the external layers of the skin – hence requiring collagen injections. If an over the counter expensive designer cream could do what it says on the box, then it would be only available on prescription and have specific instructions for the use thereof. For example, "use as directed - twice daily" because some medical creams can cause damage if applied incorrectly. In layman's terms, a cream and an ointment are two very different things. There is a significant difference; an ointment is stronger.

To explain what wrinkles really are and how they are formed.
Muscle tension causes a dominant muscle to literally get stuck in a groove and deflect the collagen. Overtime the muscle has been used more than the other muscles and therefore, become the strongest. The surrounding muscles by lack of use have become weaker. All facial muscles need to be worked to prevent this dominance and allow the muscles to relax. Unwittingly, BOTOX® toxin has become a friend of facial exercise as it artificially achieves the same result.

To highlight the inappropriate language and sales techniques used by the cosmetic enhancement businesses.
One term bantered around is a "non –invasive procedure." but if that procedure involves a needle that punctures the skin it is invasive. Cosmetic Surgery is a business, make no mistake, and just like any other business; it only survives by having repeat business, new products and are in business to make a profit. They have sales and a marketing department with call centres, team leaders, managers and a prepared script to sell you a procedure or treatment. They are employed to try to sell you something, a dream. They have targets to reach and can even make an extra commission by offering you a financial plan!

A behind-the-scenes documentary at the UK's largest cosmetic procedure provider Transform, turning over £40 million per annum.
http://www.channel4.com/programmes/bums-boobs-and-BOTOX®

To remind everyone to be natural.
That "Mother Nature" knows best - the science behind -exercising facial muscles. Aging is aging, even after many facelifts older celebrities STILL look their age. Sadly perhaps some actually look older than they should? Going to the spa to have treatments with skin creams will help; the creams boast circulation which is exactly what facial exercise does; i.e. it increases circulation to bring the essential nutrients supplied by the blood, not the cream, to the structures of the face.

Fitface's secondary mission

To alter the public's current mindset that cosmetic treatments by needles or knives are both quick and easy.
Unnatural facial "procedures" are not painless, and not without risks and not without unpleasant side effects (even for the wallet)! They are also beginning to divide women socially; between normally critical-thinking women and sheep as well as economically between the have's and the have not's.

They all make the face swell and bruise; this is unnatural. The body is trying desperately to heal the abuse. Many thousands of women suffer minor side effects such as headaches. Others have worse problems such as lumps, and a few suffer permanent disfigurement and loss of nerve function. Some more unlucky souls do acquire brain damage, others die. Not only, it isn't worth the risk, but ultimately you will age faster than if you did nothing at all except Fitface because its non invasive hands free facial toning.

To change the public's attitudes from the current separation of face and body when it comes to exercising; towards an understanding that exercise does not stop at the neck.
It really is madness to think that blood (which carries life itself to the cells in the form of essential nutrients and oxygen) stops circulating at the base of the neck! Face muscles actually work

just below the surface of facial skin and need stimulation and the same essential nutrients as the rest of the body.

In the past, there was not such a separation of face and body as proven by the American "Godfather of Fitness" Jack LaLanne http://www.zimbio.com/Alfredo+Lalanne/articles/hCVa3nzm9u2/Jack+LaLanne+Died+Fitness+King+Dies+Age+96

To supply information on facial anatomy as well as explain the physiology workings of the skin.
To describe facial anatomy in easily understandable medical terms, the functions of the multiple layers of the skin, tissues and muscles and to illustrate how the physiology of the skin works together in conjunction with the body's natural systems.

Therefore; each layer requires a different treatment - no one solution is perfect for all. Hence over the counter skin creams do not work as well as purported. At best, they are superficial for the outer skin layer which is dead! Remember that between 30,000 and 40,000 dead skin cells fall off your body every hour! Therefore topical creams are ineffectual except as superficial moisturisers.
http://health.howstuffworks.com/skin-care/information/anatomy/shed-skin-cells.htm

To reveal the truth behind the meaning of clinical trials.
Some scientific test results on anti-aging products are not fully revealed and the meaning of the data is camouflage to "package" and sell the merchandise.

For example: A legitimate study may be carried out on a moisturiser and the test results conclusively prove that the product works. But the negative side effect, that the body stops producing emollients (natural skin moisturiser) is not revealed. Mother Nature stops producing what it does not need (as it was artificially introduced). However, when the artificial cream is not applied; it takes the body's natural skin systems inner biological processes 28 days to fully respond. Because nature takes time to recovery from unnatural intervention a customer, having bought such a cream will notice a dry skin and (mislead) buys more cream!

- A legitimate claim may be made about a product but the information concerning the adverse effects on the face is quashed.
- A face cream may work well under the microscope or in trials but in practice, the body's natural mechanisms shut down and stop working to compensate.

To alert the public to the s real side-effects of BOTOX®.
Like the inability to communicate with new-born infants and the distressed caused to the child. Furthermore, to disclose the enormous funds that are put aside by Allergan to bury lawsuits that are settled out of court as just a necessary expense of doing business.
http://en.wikipedia.org/wiki/Allergan

To adjust men's attitudes to facial exercise.
Jack LaLanne was possibly the first American person to recognize the benefits of facial exercise. He was very into body building and knew that face exercise naturally prevents wrinkles and folds on the face. Interestingly, he is also a testament to my theory that facial exercise is, in addition, good for the sense organs and hair.

Perhaps men are more receptive to new ideas or do understand the fundamental principles of exercise. I say this because the first book I sold at a seminar was to a man in his 70's. I am not certain, but I think he was there with his wife, although the book was for him.
http://www.jacklalanne.com/jacks-adventures/firsts.php

To build self-esteem and to value self.
By tearing down the celebrity image myth, to show vulnerable young teenagers that the pictures are untrue, therefore unobtainable. It is all a multimillion pound illusion, designed to make money by creating an artificial need that cannot be satisfied.

To enable all people to work positively with what they have been given naturally.
Facial exercise works for all people and the results show. To teach face exercises and demonstrate that there is another way to go, rather than to be stuck on a merry go round of trying to achieve the impossible and become depressed by expectations.

Ultimate Fitface mission

To change the image of facial exercise.

In the meantime:

To save a few souls.
From either getting on the merry-go-round of going "under the knife" or from having them injected with poisons or fillers. There is another way with better results – Fitface!

To make Fitface a brand with a skin care range.
The choice for real natural beautiful, from the inside out with face exercise classes at beauty salons or spas and gyms all over the world teaching people to embrace and enhance what they were born with. Together with a natural, fragrance free pH balanced light moisturiser, a hydration spray, exfoliation wipes and another moisturiser for mature skins. I wish, I hope, I dream.

To produce a series of Fitface DVDs.
I have not (thus far) as the stop/start/pause facilities of such a DVD can be frustrating when learning. Currently, I feel that a book or cards are the best. However, this is probably because I don't know anything else or how to produce one!

To incorporate Fitface within a known exercise routine to make a new all over body and face brand.
Or perhaps to be as an extra addition to a program as the warm up or the cool down to all exercise programs?

To find a celebrity who cares enough about the lack of body confidence (and the epidemic of body dysmorphia) in young people to promote Fitface to encourage natural beauty
Perhaps there is one who puts health before beauty?

To remind the world that ultimately we love people for their insides not their outsides!
We love those who we love, regardless of their looks.

To make aging gracefully okay.
We all will age – no one escapes it and only the very, very few (in the short term don't look their age), but it does and will catch up

with them with a vengeance! Ageing is natural, as you get older other health issues will and do take over, unless you are very, very lucky. In the meantime, you can have a youthful lovely skin and do Fitface to prevent premature aging.

Fitface vision

To reverse the Western world's attitudes as to what makes us look beautiful, likeable or successful.
We all really know that it is the inside that counts but we (including me) are still fixated on external beauty! Men are more fixated on money because with it brings "power", a sense of being King of the Jungle and with it, the ability to buy what they think they want, from a beautiful appendage/arm candy or beautiful things like a collection of wonderful paintings.

It is such a strange a phenomenon, that we, the public, who ought to be so intelligent has "bought into" such lunacy. As one man once crudely said to me, "When you happen to see a strikingly beautiful tall slim woman, on the arm of a short fat ugly man; you do not wonder why she is with him; but you do wonder why he is the only man in the room who doesn't want to "f …her." I got his point, ultimately beauty is skin deep.

However, my vision is flawed, because if I were to achieve it, then the world would be a much poorer place; humans would only be concerned with ultimate self survival - dependent on the kindness of others, (as in a world war or major natural global disaster). Moreover, even today in remote places, life skills are the pinnacle of success, when one is forced back to nature the strongest still "gets the girl" so strong is our DNA.

History of Fitface

I grew up in England the really fat, unmercifully teased (bullied) ugly duckling but after losing tons of weight in my mid teens (well I had a crush on the local doctor who had put me on a diet) I had blossomed. However, a few pounds plus went on, and I could never be described as skinny being called everything from "you look well fed" by an admiring Greek boyfriend to having a Rubenesque figure, plump or curvy. My only exercise was on the dance floor, flaunting – some would say from a repressed convent education – perhaps?

In my early twenties (over 30 years ago – early 1980's) I met my new man (a Mexican American) who was obsessed with keep fit/muscles; to me he was gorgeous. He forced me to work out (which I hated at first), and I lost tons of weight. Trimmed and toned up I thought that I looked amazing and felt wonderful.

A little later my ex-partner wanted a facelift, be him only 30 or 31 (I can't remember). He was feeling down, (we were still sort of friends), and I thought it was a good idea. My selfish reasoning was that if he looked better he would get a new girlfriend and get over me. We talked to the surgeons (the best money could buy) and we both thought it was going to be a simple procedure, just in and out and a few days later he would look like a different person – handsome. Were we naïve? "Yes, most definitely and so now, I don't want the same to happen to you!"

Cutting a long story short, sadly for him, it was not simple. After all it was radical surgery, i.e. cutting out healthy tissue, plus it was early days for cosmetic surgery, so he was left with a botched job; **he looked horrendous**. I felt terrible, responsible, and guilty – I had encouraged him!

His whole face had been yanked up behind his ears and he was left with a clump of hair on the top of his head like the Pope's cap. The surgeon had said that he had been "difficult" and that they pulled back and cut out more skin away than normal. My ex was naturally bruised; bloodied and battered but far more than we expected. However, we both thought that things would calm down in time. They did try to "fix things" but he never looked normal again. Admittedly, the numbness down one side of his face subsided eventually but when I saw him for the last time (some 15 years after the operation) he said the tightness remained and he still regretted the whole episode.

That early experience had put paid to any ideas I might ever have had, then or later, about having any facial surgery.

Soon afterwards I saw and bought a book about facial exercises; I knew exercise was good for the body; I had never looked better, so I reasoned that it must also be good for the face. I tried a few but without instant results stuck it in a drawer. Young I did not reason that as with body exercises (that I had been doing for a couple of years) I wanted instance results. I had a life to lead, What with a job, body exercises, makeup, clubbing and parties, I didn't have time – besides, I thought I looked great – who needed it? To be fair I probably didn't. I was young, a vegetarian and loved to exercise, but I also liked booze and the sun (still do)!

Some years later, in my early thirties I began to notice that I had developed a few fine lines under my eyes; a couple of crow's feet and the beginnings of dips and sags. I looked "tired," my skin just wasn't as radiant as it was in my youth and I noticed the emergence of a double chin. Not liking what I saw in the mirror; I remembered the book that I had brought with me from America (I was now living in England) about facial exercises.

"Hands free" development

I began the exercise routine in earnest, with complete dedication and to my amazement, it worked; I looked rejuvenated. Being of an obsessive nature; I have subsequently tried almost every facial exercise technique available, bought all the gadgets, watched endless videos and read countless medical books. They all taught me something, even the bad methods taught me what to avoid, as they say, practice makes perfect.

Originally, the main thing I noticed was that some **exercises used the hands, and some others did not.** I was curious, and I wondered why? It didn't make sense to me, either in all the exercises, one needed to use your hands, or in none. The more I read, the more fascinated I became. I discovered that (in simple terms) most of the facial muscles are connected to the underside of the skin. And many in turn either to each other or they worked together, in simple terms like an intricate web across the face attached to the underside of the skin.
http://en.wikipedia.org/wiki/Facial_muscles

Therefore, to me using the hands could potentially (and in practice most probably would) stretch the overlying skin far too much; certainly more than nature intended. Moreover, since Elastin (the protein that makes skin stretchy/elastic) **stops being built at puberty – I reasoned that I had better not damage it**! Facial exercise was in its infancy in the Europe and not knowing any differently (and half-listening to my mother who told me not "**rub in**" face cream every night I decided to err on the side of caution and only to do those exercises that were "hand-free."

I can only speak from over twenty-five years of personal experience; they worked and continue to work for me. **My skin has not been pulled beyond what it could be naturally**. "Hands-free" is the way for me; it is the logical choice, especially now that I am far more knowledgeable and know what lies beneath the skin, but I will not bore you with a mass of medical jargon, or I will never get to the point of Fitface – the book on face and neck exercises.

I continued to practice and noticed that some exercises worked better than others. Moreover, I noticed that in some exercises I was told to "hold" the muscle and in others, I was asked to rapidly work the muscle. I knew the different between many repetitions and static movement (no movement – holding steady) but I didn't know why or what was happening. In other words, which should I be doing for the best? I didn't even know the names let alone what was happening! (See Chapter 3 for a further explanation).

- **Isotonic** (meaning same tension)
- **Isometric** (meaning same distance or not moving)
- **Isokinetic** (meaning same speed)

Still curious, I wanted to get to the bottom of it. I searched and searched for more information on facial muscles and how they really, REALLY worked with endless visits to the library (no internet in those days). My research was only possible by ploughing through expensive medical books and journals (that I had ordered to read). To my amazement, despite the vast amount of research undertaken, there were still no absolute conclusive answers that everyone agreed upon.

I learned masses, about the anatomy of the face, how the overlying skin functions and most importantly how muscles grow. (See Chapter 3 for a further explanation).

- **Muscle hypertrophy** increase in muscle cell size
- **Muscle hyperplasia** increase in muscle cell numbers

I combined all my knowledge and experience and began to perfect some of my ideas. I experimented on myself and with friends until I was satisfied that I had found the answer to easily obtaining and maintaining a toned glowing healthy-looking face for a lifetime. I wanted the exercises to be fun, fast, and easy to do, to learn and be performed at any time, in any place.

My main focus was that The Fitface technique was to be designed to be natural; with no over stretching or pulling of the face by the hands. Therefore all the exercises are performed "hands free" so as not to put any unnecessary pressure on the delicate facial tissues - that is the real message in Fitface.

Once I was completely satisfied that I had perfected some basic exercises, (which took me over twenty years) I decided to put pen to paper and write my first book. To make my book a comprehensive analysis of the benefits of facial exercise, I also conducted more research and included information on the alternative natural and unnatural beauty products available. Two years later I published the first Fitface.

Fitface book's publication history

I started writing Fitface in about 2006 at my desk when I was working part-time in the marketing suites of various new homes developers. Sometimes one didn't see a customer for days. The job is very different to the plush marketing suites in the USA where the idea (I believe) is to sell as many upgrades as possible. Here it is more management and less selling of frills, sometimes there are none available, its literally house type A, B or C.

I decided to take 6 months off and finish it in Florida which I did.

Book 1- 2008
Fitface: The natural face-lift
The Guide to Fun Facial Toning Exercises

This was my first attempt at a book and it is sad to say that there were too many typing and spelling errors, things that were not fully explained and there were no photographs. I am pleased to report that it is out of print.

In the next edition I obviously wanted to correct my mistakes, to make it more comprehensive and to add photographs.

Book 2- 2010
Fitface: The natural face-lift
Hands Free Facial Toning Exercises
http://www.amazon.com/Fitface-ebook/dp/B0049H9538
http://www.amazon.com/Fitface-Hands-Facial-Toning-Exercises/dp/1453777830

My second book was and is a totally comprehensive guide to Fitface "hands free" exercise complete with a full history of Fitface conception, my thoughts and philosophies. A definitive guide on "How and why" you should exercise your face, notably "hands free" with over 60 Fitface face and neck exercises.

Fitface is divided into two parts for easy reading. The first half is all about information, my background and, "why and how" facial exercise rejuvenates your face. The second half shows you "how to do Fitface hands free" facial toning with photographs and instructions."

Part 1
Why Fitface?
It is educational and informative. Fitface takes you back to the basics, to explore the science behind facial skin, focusing on facial muscles, illustrated with where they are in the face and how they work. And covers why we age and how to prevent it.

Fitface takes a no-nonsense in depth look at the alternatives to facial exercises – namely needles or knives and answers all the really important questions like "Where does BOTOX® really go to?" "Will I scar from a facelift?" "Can I die from a facelift?" "What if something goes wrong?"

Charlotte delves into the myths of the billion dollar industry of cosmeceuticals and explains why some (most) non prescription cosmetic creams don't work, can't work and won't work; as well as a look into the world of the weird and wacky from - skull lifts to vitamin IV's - which are all the rage in Japan. Fitface touches on celebrity images and motivates you to think positively about your own self image.

Part 2
Fitface programs
This is where the serious fun and work begins, the exercise routines. Fitface motivates and guides you through the 3 step program starting with the easy Fitface basic routine. Each step takes you further, to more advanced exercises. You will learn over 60 new exercises ALL with photographs and easy instructions to guide you through.

There are four routines in total ranging in difficulty from beginner to advanced student. In no time at all Fitface face exercises will become second nature to you and both you and your friends will notice the change.

Many chapters are summarized at the end of each chapter and in the very last chapter, "How to maintain a healthy lifestyle is summed up in the Final Words.

Lastly, but by no means least there are hundreds of references at the back of the book for you, if you feel so inclined, to research further into the world of facial fitness, surgery or any other of the subjects covered.

Book 2 Oct 2010 updated ISBN: 978 0615422442
This book is distributed in the UK and Europe with only limited availability in the USA. It is almost exactly the same Fitface book as above - only better! An editor corrected all the silly spelling and grammatical mistakes (there are still a few) and perhaps I added a line or two, I should remember, but don't!!

Book 2 (The supplementary book) **- Fitface Foundations 2011**

This book is simply a supplementary book containing just the instructions, facial exercises and photographs - taken directly from book 2 part 2 of Fitface: The natural face-lift. Hands Free Facial Toning Exercises

Fitface Foundations

http://www.barnesandnoble.com/w/fitface-foundations-charlotte-hamilton/1104547730
http://www.amazon.com/Fitface-Foundations-ebook/dp/B005LB7XZ8/ref=sr_1_1?ie=UTF8&qid=1336645891&sr=8-1

Fitface Foundations is an excellent additional book to purchase later. It has more and different exercises to those contained here within. Keeping fresh with exercises will motivate you and exercise every muscle in your face (which I can never stress enough it is so important).

Book 3 - 2012
Fitface facial exercises
The book on face and neck exercises

You are reading it now!

What most men and women want to know is how to look their best forever. So if you do not care about "How" or "Why" facial exercise works just skip to the face and neck exercises. But, if you need or want to know why, then PLEASE, please read this entire book.

Here within I have tried not to lecture or labour on too much about what happens where and when one exercises the face. The key, salient point is that if you want a fresh, toned glowing face and to prevent wrinkles from getting hold of your face earlier than you want them to, then you must give your face the same attention that you give your body. Exercise and eat right. Your face just like your body works from the inside out. - be you, a man or a woman.

Most of the essential physiological information was in the last book (Book 2). I have updated much of that information and included additional information that perhaps should have been in the other book. I have focused the information sections on the new developments in the health and beauty industry, to include new fangled thinking, innovative ideas and the latest alternative products available.

I have listened to your comments and emails, and my newly designed exercises are current, targeted to today's 'quick and easy to do' world, especially bearing in mind the younger generation, whom I hope to attract. I believe that a key issue in staying youthful is starting early to develop good lifetime practices, be it diet or exercise. Good habits produce strong neurological pathways to the brain that last a lifetime.

Life moves at such an incredible speed that what I wrote about in book 2 has now been superseded by new developments. Everyday science is progressing; there are medical discoveries and new cosmetic procedures to bring to the market. The beauty industry changes too. There are new conceptions of beauty, a new look and alongside them comes a range of new products to enter the market place.

People's attitudes too change with time, especially social acceptability of artificial techniques to retard the aging process. They have become more socially acceptable. However, their acceptability has brought forward more concerns regarding their long-term use. Most worryingly of all are their addictive qualities and consequently the dependency trends. Moreover, such concentration on "looks" is leading to increased problems with children from body dysmorphic syndrome. (The person complains of a defect in either one feature or several features of their body; or vaguely complains about their general appearance, which causes psychological distress that causes clinically significant distress or impairs occupational or social functioning).
http://en.wikipedia.org/wiki/Body_dysmorphic_disorder

So much so, that there are campaigns such as Body Confidence Campaign. The government has convened a group of experts to identify non-legislative solutions to tackle the causes of low levels of body confidence.
http://www.homeoffice.gov.uk/equalities/equality-government/body-confidence/

And - AnyBody being established to teach children that it is okay to look the way they are made naturally.

Times are changing, and I am here in this book trying to address some of the issues of our changing world of beauty. Men and women are so busy in today's world that they do not have time to investigate issues fully and believe what they see in the pages of beauty magazines and read in the newspapers. Both sexes have complete and utter trust in their doctors;, they are beyond reproach we hope like our politicians. However, unlike our politicians (hopefully) they are in business to make an income for their families and they will only remain in business if they make a profit. Furthermore, in England I believe I am right in saying that the Law on our National Health system has recently changed and that each doctor's practise is now considered an independent business providing a service.

Today, cosmetic surgery practices make no secret that they are generating enormous profits and are proud to have many locations. Their sales advisors are highly trained, the best in the business and these days can offer finance plans. As with any sale one must ask oneself what is in it for them? The answer is of course "money." You are as naïve as I was in my twenties if you think you will walk into the doctor's office and he would say, "Young lady, I think you should think twice about what you are asking me to do, as you are only XYZ years old." But actually, that was exactly, what had happened to me over 30 years ago.

Allergan, the manufacturers of BOTOX® have grown from strength to strength despite the number of lawsuits and out of court settlements. In 2002, BOTOX® was born; with FDA approval. In 2004, Allergan achieved $2 billion in sales and by 2006, $3 billion in sales. But on February 8, 2008, the FDA announced that BOTOX® has "been linked in some cases to adverse reactions, including respiratory failure and death, due to its ability to spread to areas distant from the site of the injection." In April 2009, the FDA updated its mandatory boxed warning cautioning that the effects of botulinum toxin type A may spread from the area of injection to other areas of the body, causing symptoms similar to those of botulism. Despite this Allegan continues to prosper. The whole push sales strategy story of phenomenal incentives to doctors, cut throat business dealings, and shenanigans makes compelling reading. For example, Allergan's profit plunged in 2010 after it agreed to pay $600 million for promoting BOTOX® as a treatment for headaches and other uses for which it had not been approved.
http://en.wikipedia.org/wiki/Allergan

I remain as passionate as ever about the subject matter that I write on; eating correctly, body and face exercises (for the facial muscles to remain looking toned for life). Why stop exercising at the neck? For me, it is a "no brainer" and makes complete common sense. However, it's an uphill battle, because the cosmeceuticals (cosmetic products with biologically active ingredients purporting to have medical or drug-like benefits), pharmaceutical, spas and cosmetic surgery businesses are all able to publish adverts and editorials about complete and utter rubbish on 'How to stay youthful looking' I sometimes feel like doing the same! If I were to do likewise, and endorsed a cream or product, saying, "use this" and it will do what facial exercise does; then I might become a wealthy woman! But could I look myself in the mirror? At 18 years old yes, now um, I'm not so sure? *Who am I kidding? Of course I would, we can all be bought, regrettably.*

Reading platforms

Books were once only available in print. Within just 5 years (when I started publishing) I have seen an unprecedented rise in eBooks purchases. In 2010 print equalled eBooks. My last statistical information was that as of Christmas 2011 and eBook sales outsold print. Therefore, I have made the whole book more eBook friendly with more salient facts and faster access to relevant links.

I once again decided not to produce a DVD. Mainly, because I need some serious help in producing one, plus the exercises here within are so simple it's almost an unnecessary encumbrance. Because you need to practice each face exercise at your own pace and not to have to keep up with a set pace as in body movement's routine. Nevertheless, I would still like to, still, there is always YouTube – (which I must remember to do).

Information

In this book, I have directly sourced much of the information from the internet in order that you the reader **believe me** that facial exercises do work and the reasons why the alternatives don't last. Yes, there is some bad and misleading information out there which I have tried to correct. Some even written by my competition! Although, to be fair, medical science is in its infancy and we are learning, but in reality we haven't really got a clue. We can't cure the common cold, cancer, HIV, etc. We are still light-years away from having a magic wand that we could waft over a patient and receive an instant diagnosis (as to their condition) as featured in Star Trek by Dr. McCoy. Like me, he believed in less intrusive treatments and the body's innate recuperative powers. Perhaps one-day science fiction will become science fact and we could simply touch a wound to induce healing like an alien being.

I have reduced some of the subject matter and depth of knowledge offered in this edition of Fitface as most new readers wanted to "cut to the chase" and do the exercises. Book 2 Fitface Hands-free facial toning exercises remains a good initial basic source for information. However, for those equally interested in what happens anatomically and scientifically I have left in references and links for further research. If you do nothing else, I strongly urge you to take an in-depth look at where the muscles are under the skin and see how they interact to form facial expressions, I would highly recommend these websites:

Muscles of Facial Expression
Anatomy Tutorial
http://www.youtube.com/watch?v=Xmz3oLrnzBw
Artnatomy
Anatomical basis of facial expression learning tool
http://www.artnatomia.net/uk/index.html

Exercises and routines in Book 3

50 face exercises (mainly different from Book 2).
11 completely new routines, designed to take under 10 minutes.

All the daily routines are short, sharp, effective and easy to learn.
Five routines - concentrate on **specific areas** of the face and neck

1. Whole face
2. Mouth Lower face – (Chin, jaw line jowls)
3. Eyes
4. Mouth Upper face – (Nasolabial folds/cheeks)
5. Neck

Six routines - concentrate on a **combination** of the 5 areas of the face and neck exercises.

Plus a warm up and cool down program within the 10 minutes!

You can either incorporate the 10-minute routines in with your normal body exercise workout as part of your warm up or as part of your cool down or use as a standalone program.

Glossary and references

People have less and less time to read. Bearing that in mind, coupled with the fact that publishing methods keep changing and evolving with new apps and technologies, I've tried something new. Instead of putting the glossary and reference section at the back of the book I've included them in the body of the text, where, in my opinion, I believe they belong.

Why? I hear you say. Well, to save you time looking up words that you are unsure of in a normal glossary and to satisfy the copyright of the original author of the reference material or direct quote to which I am referring in my overview or writings.

Spelling and grammar

I am English but having spent approximately 15 years of my adult life in the USA which translated means that I speak and write American too! However, I have decided to go back to my roots (a sign of my age) and write this book with the aid of a British spell check and English grammar. Therefore, some things may appear "Mickey Mouse" to my friends across the pond or odd here in England as well!

Please bear in mind that this was in no way intended to be a literary giant and in that vein, I apologize in advance for breaking with some tradition prose rules for brevity as well as spelling/punctuation mistakes or typos. Feel free to be my editor and email in my errors.

Printing

Standard paperback paper is getting thinner and thinner. Therefore, for those reading my book in print, I have decided to print each photograph on a new, separate page on the right-hand side of the book. Additionally, this gives you a place to write your notes.

Personal observations

Times have and are changing and I must confess that my preaching the benefits of facial exercise has been helped recently by a change in attitudes; swinging towards the benefits of facial exercise and away from needles and knives. Journalists are beginning to see the long term results of stars incessant preoccupation with constant facelifts and BOTOX® injections and now the results are not pretty. For example, an article entitled **"Ageless? It's so ageing, Darling"** I used to envy the Women Who Did It, but now we're the ones having the last laugh. And to hell with the laughter lines!
Written by - Mimi Spencer of You Magazine.
March 2012.The Sunday supplement of the Daily Mail.
http://www.dailymail.co.uk/home/you/article-2111494/Ageless-It-s-ageing-darling.html#ixzz1qVDt7ksy

Accompanying the article, there was a tragic picture of Brook Shields, Daryl Hannah and Melanie Griffith. As they all look that bad collectively in the photograph, then goodness knows what they look like in the flesh at home!

The cosmetics industries are changing too, seeking new customers in the East; they are developing new products - nutircosmetics (see Chapter 4) and campaigns designed to appeal to the Chinese market that have for generations had faith in Chinese medicine and facial exercises. They are compulsory in Chinese schools (mandatory twice daily). It is a big step in the right direction towards universal acknowledgement that exercise doesn't stop at the shoulders!
Chinese Eye Exercises at Beijing No. 2 School
www.youtube.com/watch?v=ol4H0oP9xwA&feature=related
Chinese little girl - Doing Chinese Eye Exercise
www.youtube.com/watch?v=OgSbo30xaKg&feature=related
Eye Exercises
www.youtube.com/watch?v=MH3GsO9kGD4&feature=autoplay&list=PL2B1BED070825F4CB&lf=results_video&playnext=2
Chinese Eye Exercises
http://www.youtube.com/watch?v=JpToCa__HDk

Furthermore, my "facial exercise advocates/competition" has multiplied tenfold. Therefore, I must be doing something right!

Much has changed since I first sat down to write the original Fitface. Okay, it's only been 5 years in publishing terms, but I started writing about 2 years earlier which takes us back to 2006 which in terms of the acceptance of "facial exercise" was the dark ages! Then the belief was exercise forms wrinkles/folds and that I was crazy! Which I accepted as a step down from "You're mad" as it was less hurtful! Knowing I was neither mad nor crazy but that the rest of the world was (incidentally "Yes," I was told that believing that was the first sign of madness) undeterred I believed in myself.

> **Note:** The same was said to me about my having blind dates with men that I had contacted through the "Lonely Hearts Personal Adverts" when I wrote "Manhunt" - The search for Mr. Right" – now less than 20 years later there is Match.com and now it is the normal way to meet a mate!

By 2005, I had been doing facial exercises to some degree or another, on and off, with spurts of wild enthusiasm to neglecting them for months/weeks (even now I need a break) for about 20 years. There are 3 very different things between women of about my age and me:
- My forehead – lack of wrinkles or frown lines
- My nasolabial folds – only when I smile
- And the single biggest difference between me and women of my age is my neck; I have one!

Over those years, my eagerness to eradicate wrinkles and increase tone intensified, yes I was losing my looks naturally as we all do. We all age and I cannot promise you a reversal to your twenties; no one can, not BOTOX® or even the knife, only Adobe® Photoshop®! I pity the poor souls whom undergo such radical procedures, chasing the unobtainable. I have seen many of the results from death and deformity to pain and twitches ignored and overlooked by their best friends/family. Who wants to be told that they have spent a small fortune at the hands of a well meaning cosmetic surgeon, but nature didn't play ball? YES, they are left lifted, with smooth skin, a perfect taut face incapable of showing emotion and are able to overlook the new result of a weeping eye, or over sensitivity to sunlight and even an almost constant involuntary twitch at the side of the mouth. In kindness, we the friends and relatives among the knife victims overlook such minor flaws to save the "feelings" of the afflicted. It would be less outrageous if the results lasted!

I never would be so bold or so cruel as to tell my friends what I really thought – writing this perhaps I just have? But they are in such denial that they would refute my observations and not associate themselves as the target. It wasn't until recently that I really understood why I am anti surgery. I was looking at a photograph of my girlfriend with whom I had just been on holiday with and saw for the first time, the emotionless state of her face. The photograph was taken by a couple of girl backpackers when we were riding on a quad bike (all-terrain vehicles) in Panama driving down a beach-track road. We had stopped for the shot to be taken and I looked thrilled/excited/animated/joyful even with dynamic wrinkles showing and she looked "the same as always." It didn't strike me as odd at the time but at home I noticed that she was the same in all the photos, regardless of the situation!

My point being, that the flawless look says or rather communicates nothing, there is an absence of self; her face contributes nothing to her personality, but she thinks she looks great. She is so proud of her face and the fact that everyone comments that she looks just like Joan Rivers only younger (true she does) but does she not understand that Joan Rivers is a comedian and laughs about the way she looks! My friend would be horrified if she thought that anyone knew she had had a facelift or had work done yet she is the first one to suggest it to others! Why? Why not admit to surgery or BOTOX®? I am not sure? She must be on her second or even third facelift (See Chapter 4 for alternatives to face exercises and the misconceptions of what a facelift really involves). Whether or not she has surgery should not matter, yet why does it matter to her and celebrities? For her, it must be self-denial? Perhaps she is kidding herself because; she thinks that by spending money (on having herself cut up) she bought something of value. Whereas facial exercises is free and therefore, in her eyes has no value. She wants value for her hard-earned cash; furthermore, she wants the acceptance of others and for them to join her in "the expensive knife club."

Perhaps I am no different? I want you to be in my club, free from the social stigma of NOT HAVING HAD BOTOX®! Free from the knife brigade whom themselves know facelifts don't last (more than 7 - 10 years). Free to think for yourself about the risks and side effects. Free from the lies of the results. Free from the advertising media that generates adverts to entice you to buy 'stuff' to make the magazine financially viable. Free from the media propaganda showing you unrealistic Adobe® Photoshop® images of what your age group should look like (but in reality does not). Free from the pressures of looking brilliant until you die. Free to think for yourself. Fitface is free (you have already purchased the book) therefore, in today's thinking there is no value in the product. But think again, the air you breathe is free!. You do have a choice not to follow the misguided crowd.

Maybe we here in the United Kingdom are in a "Nanny State"? Maybe the citizens of the USA are beginning to feel the same? Maybe we need professionals whom are only money makers in disguise to tell us what to do, what to think and what to buy? You know that eating right and exercise are good for you. You do not need me to tell you. Knowing the truth, then surely it makes sense that exercise for the face is superior to the knife or needles? We all take things at face value, we believe we have advertising standards and we trust in our doctors. We would hate to think that a doctor would suggest surgery before exercise, but the truth is sadly different. They often have shareholders to answer to, targets to meet, staff to employ, a bottom line, another office to open, expansion plans and by generating profits, - ever more business and in a way become a victim of their own success.

Fitface was really designed by Mother Nature millions of years ago and only really modified by me. The movement of the face is natural, created to show a myriad of facial expressions in order to communicate with others. Facial expression was how we first learnt as babies to communicate with our mothers. Understanding one another allowed our ancestors to work together effectively and separated us from the animals.

Today, they still report that 94% of communication is "body language" regardless of the many technological ways we use verbal and written communication. Often just a glance of an eye says it all.

The references are from many different websites, including my competition, other facial exercise enthusiasts, beauty products manufacturers and the medical profession. If you first preview this book on the internet, I may lose you to one of those other products along the sales route, but so be it. I am very passionate in my belief in hands free facial exercise as the only real lasting method to slow the aging process of the face. I champion the cause of face exercises, and oppose fillers, particularly neurotoxins like BOTOX® and any unnecessary facial surgery such as a facelift. Therefore, unfortunately I am ingratiating myself with the media, but I am not a sheep, are you?

As much as I believe in face exercises I also believe in rest and relaxation. A body or a face constantly mentally or physically stressed is not good. The body needs time to repair and heal. Think of this like a scab, it is no good keep picking at it, or it won't heal correctly. *In other words, don't overdo it.* Don't worry if you don't get the exercises totally right. Even for me no two times that I workout my face are the same. Enjoying facial exercise and by doing so you will be building strong positive neurological connections that will develop into you wanting to exercise, just as it does with the body exercises. It is the same principal.

Photos of me growing up

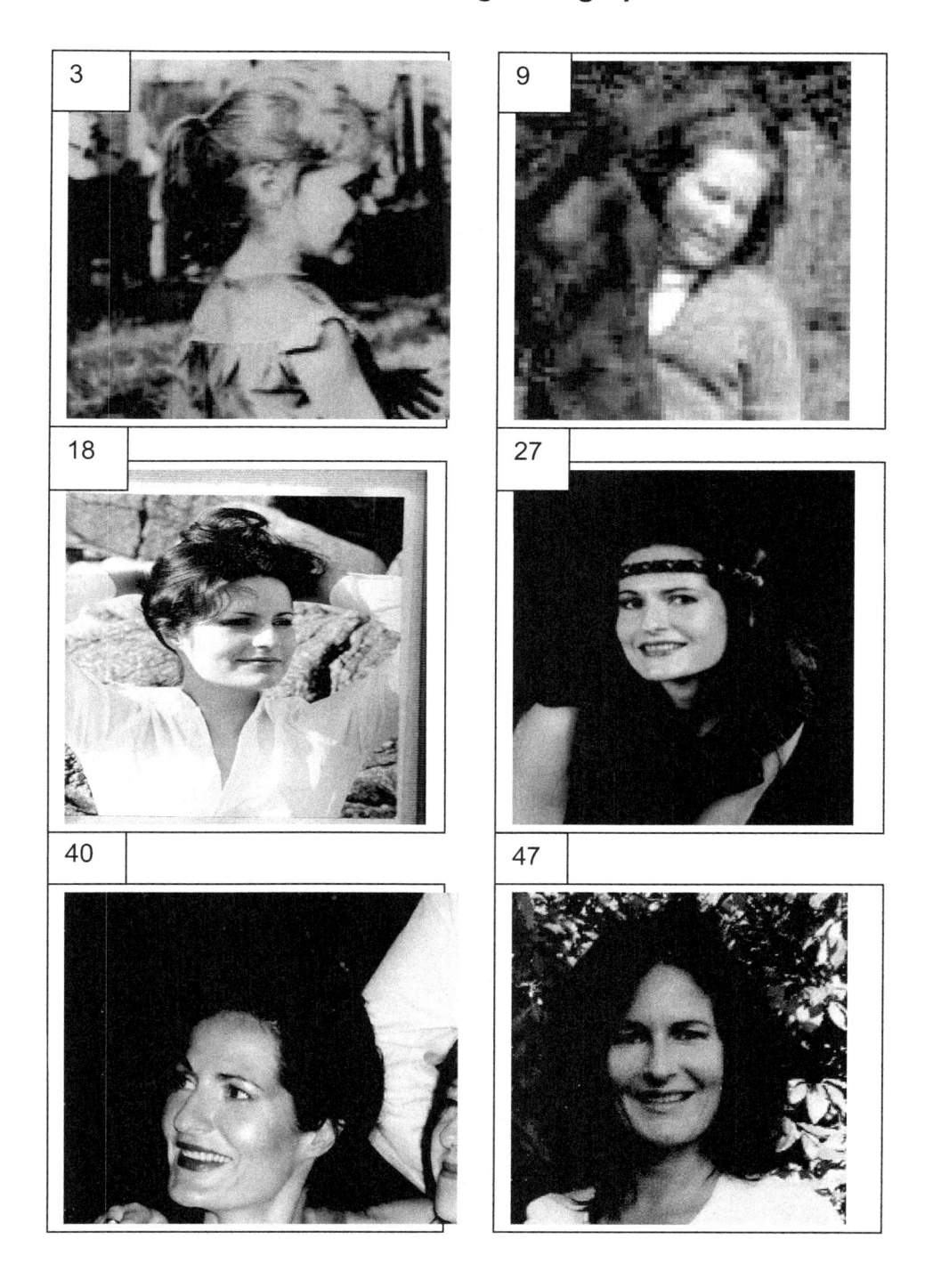

3	9
18	27
40	47

Both 54 years old

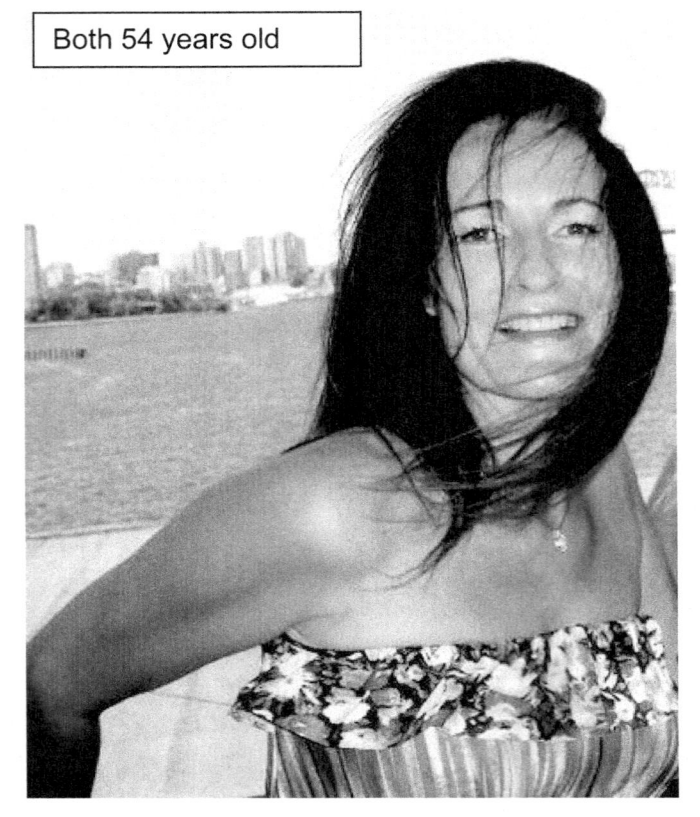

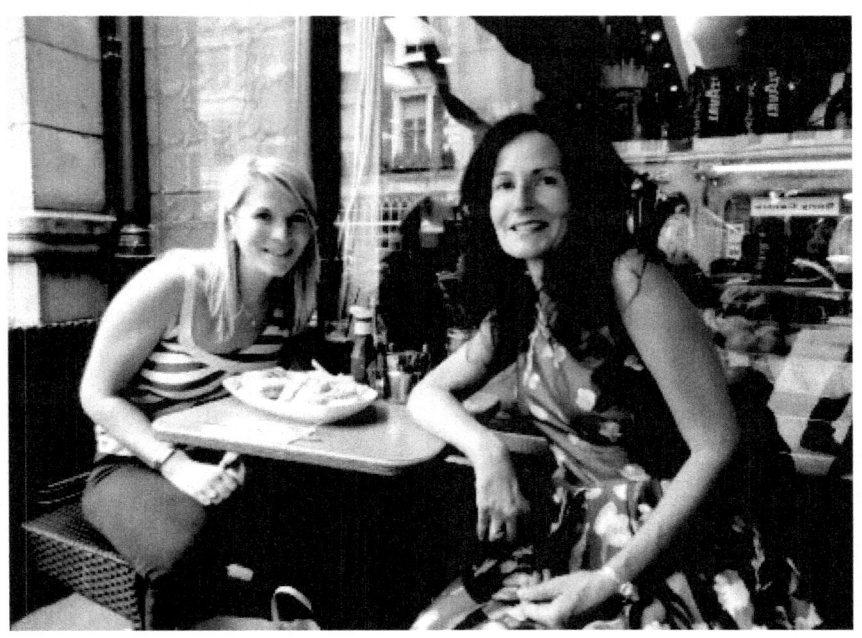

2011 aged 55

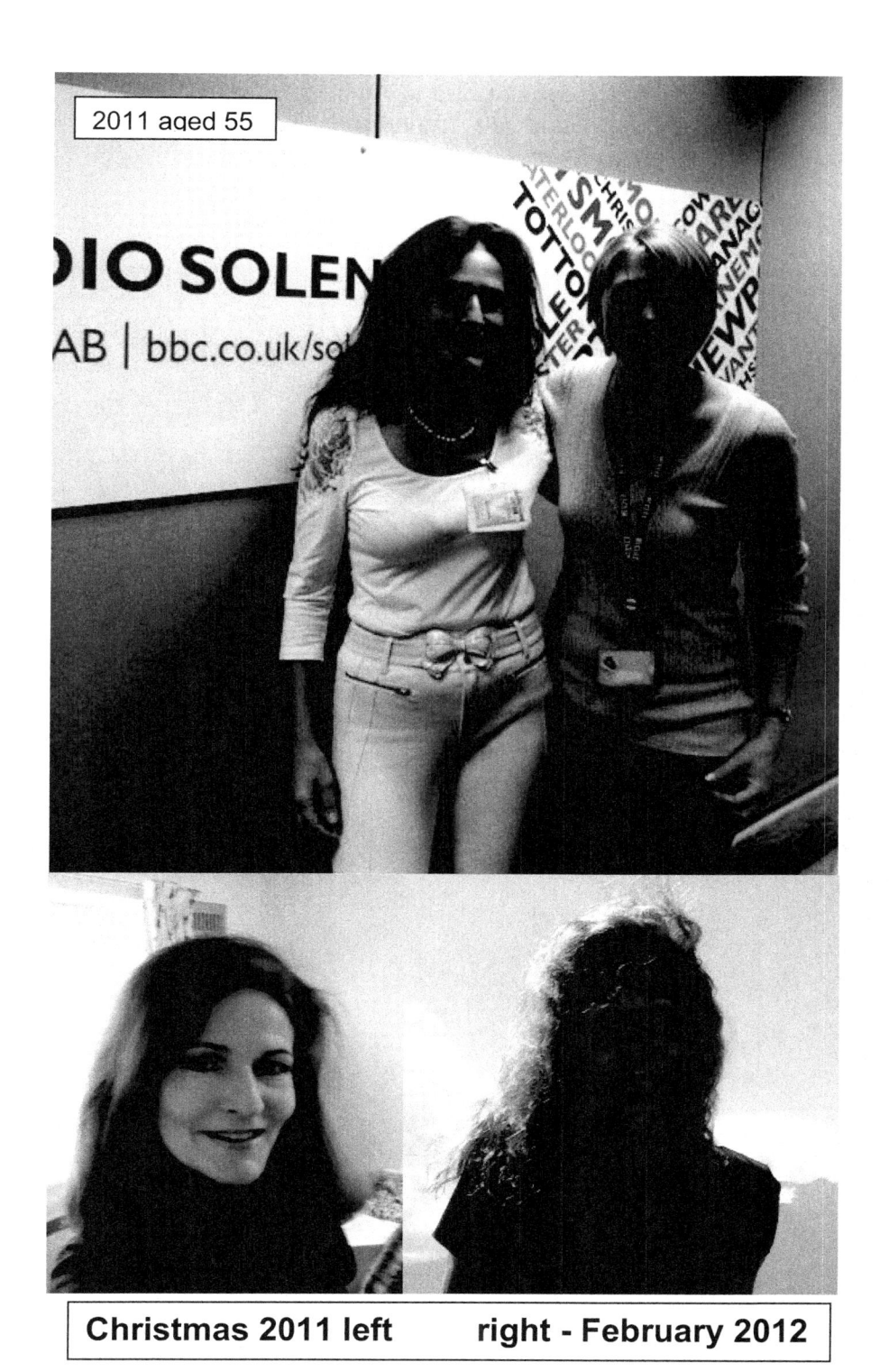

Christmas 2011 left   right - February 2012

The next few photos (before printing) were taken by my girlfriend on an ordinary camera and are untouched. We went out for a pub lunch to celebrate my coming 56th birthday (in five days time).

Considering my life of "fun andsun" I am happy with how I look..

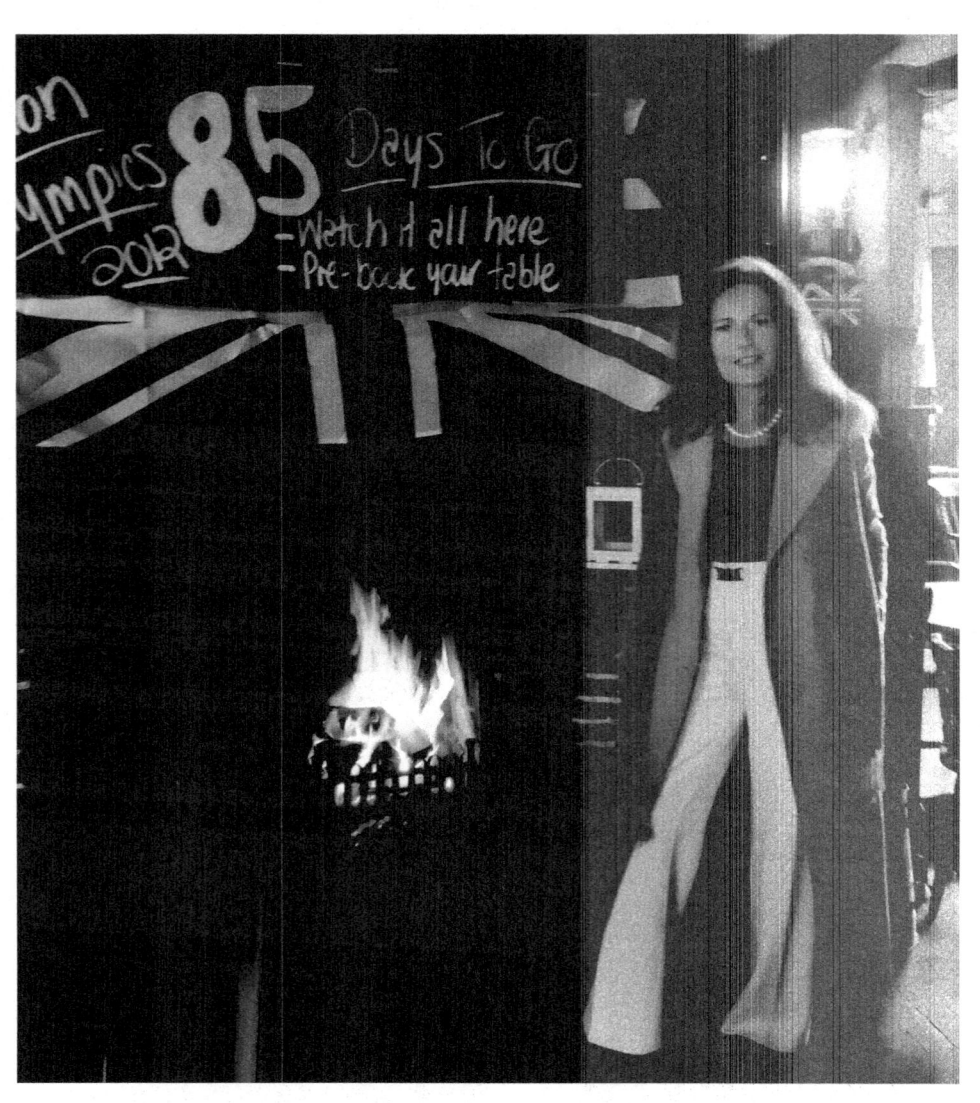

May 2nd 2012
85 days before the London Olympics

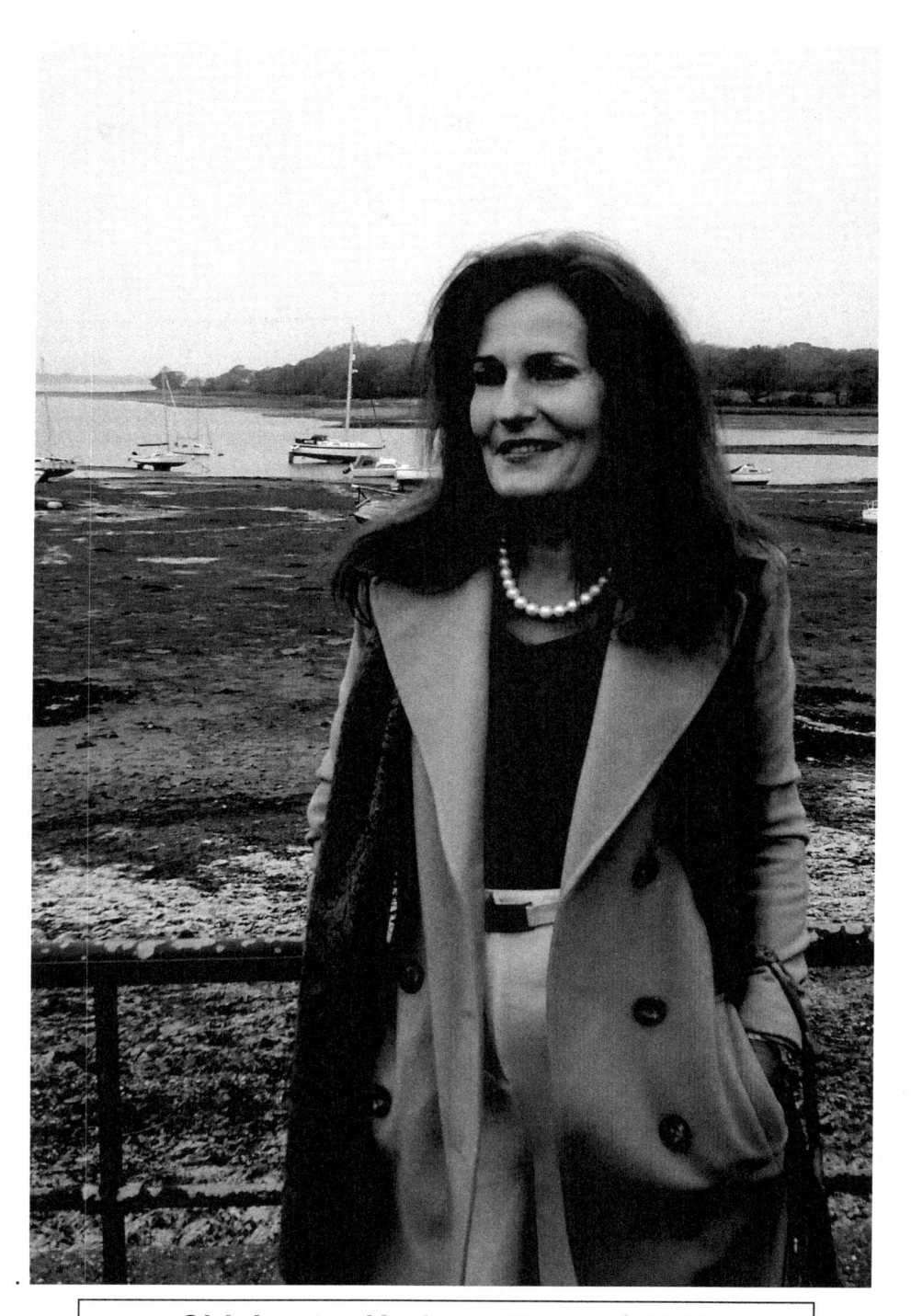

Chichester Harbour May 2nd 2012

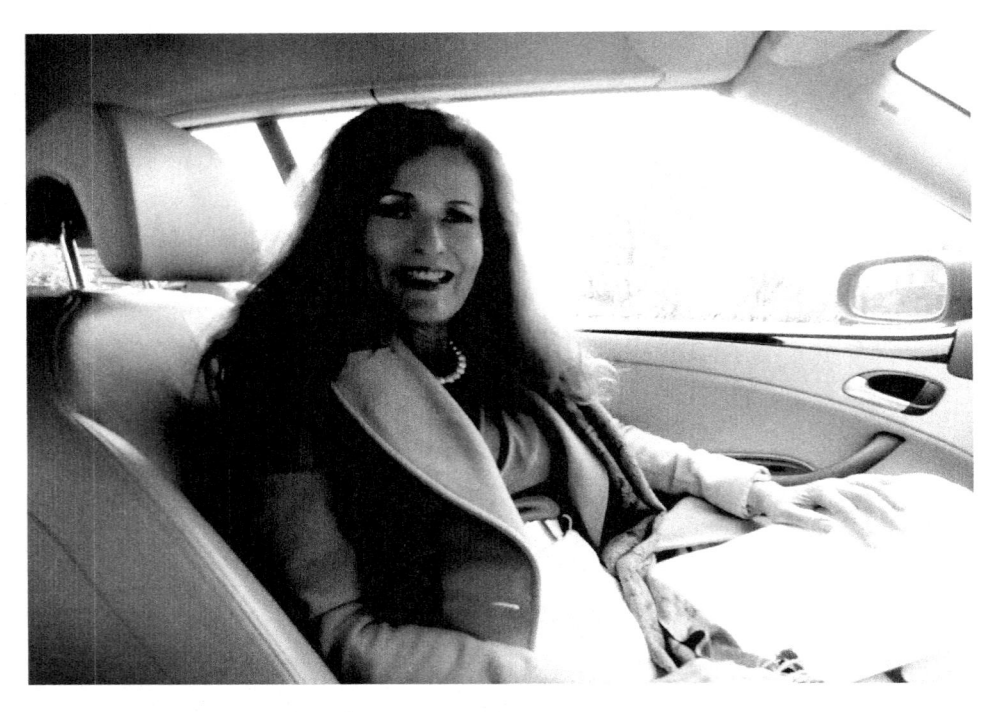

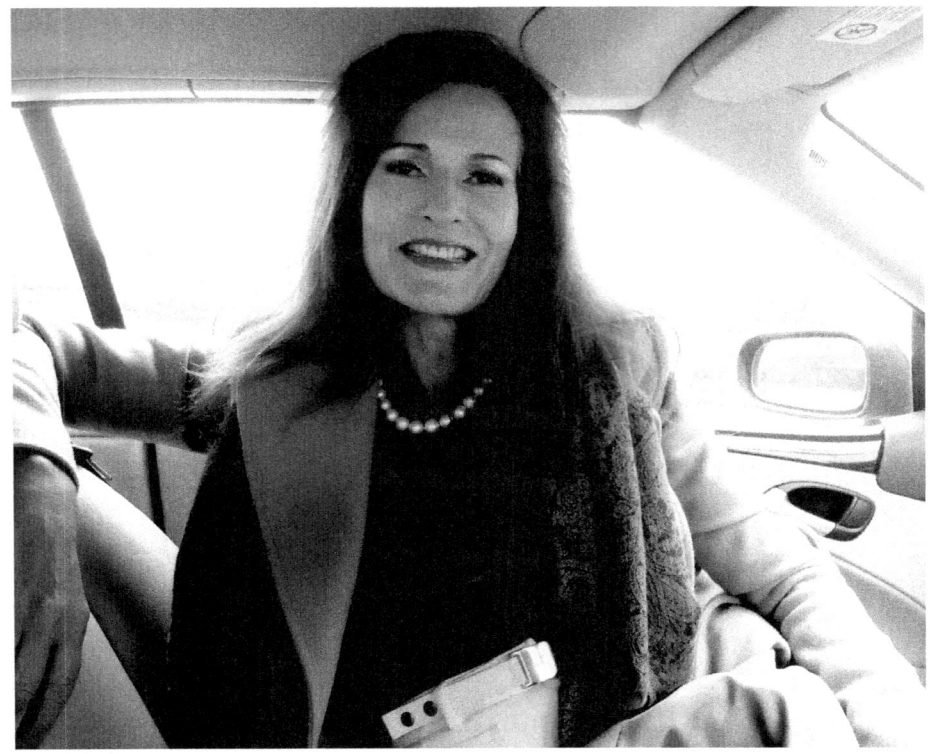

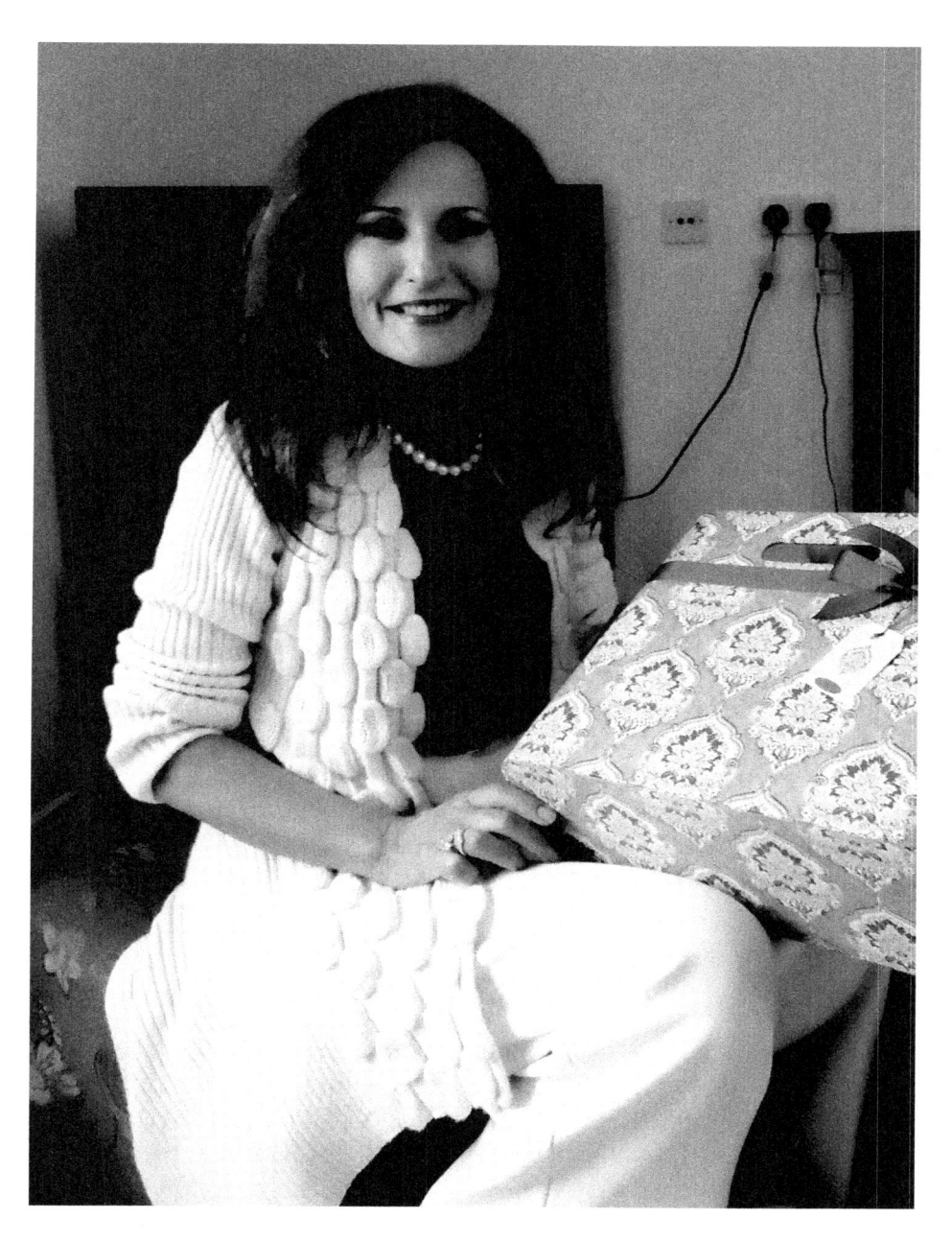

Back at home after my day out with my friend at the pub in Chichester Harbour, having just opened my birthday present (5 days early) from her.

**Fitface's techniques and methods are simple.
We all age, but Fitface puts health before beauty.
Fitface is nature's beauty spa.**

To have a fit face you must treat all layers of the face, from the inside out - especially because the outer layer is only dead cells. The skin needs a healthy internal and external environment for the face to look great.

Exercise your body and don't forget your face

For the body the extra oxygen, movement and post relaxation of muscle fibres that exercise brings is immeasurable in terms of health benefits. So why would you stop at the neck? Give your face a natural spa break by doing facial exercises - work those muscles, let them feel they way they do when you have a facial done to you at the spa. It feels good; you will look toned, fresh, and alive – why? Because you've just given your face what it wanted; extra nutrients and oxygen supplied via the blood from the extra circulation that is created by exercise.

You can achieve the same results at home naturally, exercise your face, see how feel – get the glow naturally – from exercise. At the same time, you will be blasting those potential wrinkles and unfolding stuck deflated fibrous collagen. Better still exercise actually builds collagen!

Perform facial exercises – "hands free"

Facial exercises will increase blood flow to the face/skin and facial muscles. The blood carries additional supplies of oxygen **(your face breathes internally)** and nutrients to nourish the cells. For a full explanation read Book 2 **Fitface – Hands free facial toning exercises.**

All Fitface exercises are "hands free." Your hands do not touch the face when practicing Fitface. Fitface's methods avoids over stretching of the skin. Unnatural, unnecessary pulling of the face may thin and weaken the skin causing more harm than good in the long term.

The Fitface technique totally avoids placing any excessive pressure on the face. There is no unwarranted force exerted on the face which potentially could damage the underlying elastin fibres that are responsible for the recoiling mechanism after a stress or deformation has been applied. (Elastin cannot be stimulated to grow past puberty).

Accept that aging is a natural phenomenon

It is unavoidable, just like death it will happen. Remember that the stress of worrying about it too much is far worse than the process itself - cortisol from stress is very bad for your collagen levels. Try to be as stress as free as possible in today's world!

Remember that stress is the world's biggest killer! So don't be too preoccupied with not being stressed, enjoy your life and take it as it comes.

Get adequate sleep

No one really knows exactly what happens when you sleep except that the body shuts down and puts all but essential functions to sleep, in order to rejuvenate and heal it's self. That is good enough for me!

Think positively about yourself

Remember that almost all celebrity images are "unreal," and they have been touched-up with Adobe® Photoshop® to produce nothing more than illusions and therefore - unobtainable (except with Adobe® Photoshop®)!

Do not smoke

Cigarettes significantly decrease the supply of oxygen to skin cells.

Eat and drink healthily

Water is the fuel of life.
Preservatives and additives - preserve the product but destroy you!

Keep your skin care as natural as possible

Preferably, pH balanced and to a minimum by limiting the number of products. Avoid harsh cleaners. Remember your skin care does change with age.

Let your skin breathe externally

The environment in which you live has got much to do with the condition of your skin. Inside there may be air conditioning or central heating both of which dry the face and you will not look your best. Breathe and expose your skin to fresh air. Go without wearing foundation makeup as much as you can.

Note: Be careful; yes limited sunlight is required for the production of vitamin D but don't be silly, about 20 minutes a day (although this keeps changing). A nice breeze feels fabulous and is good for you, but be sure to protect yourself from gale-force winds or you will have weather-beaten skin.

Avoid sugar

That includes alcohol (more later). Sugar destroys collagen faster and more effectively than anything else!

I have listed the above in the order of importance to me. I spent my youth enjoying life, in California, yes with smoking and drinking followed by executive stress in the UK. but I always exercised both my body and face, drank plenty – yes including wine and at 56 years of age, I do look better (or at least as good) as my friends and associates, despite some of them having had "work done" to one extent or another.

I invite you to try the Fitface face and neck facial exercises for 3 months and I can guarantee you it will work for you. Like most things "it's up to you" – for your part - you must "Just do it."

Images

I get so tired of picking up magazines with pictures of the rich and famous (like today it was Catherine Zeta Jones and Sandra Bullock – last week Kylie) and being told how I can "go for the

glow" and look just like them; if only I used this or that cream. It really is ridiculous, even if I was a fan of needles and knives my bone structure is so completely different! Worse still I only just read about Sandra Bullock's surgery.
Explaining Sandra Bullock's mystery lump
http://inyourface.ocregister.com/2011/05/04/explaining-sandra-bullocks-mystery-lump/28927
Just seen Catherine Zeta Jones before and after pictures
http://famousplastic.com/gallery/celebrity-botox/#!prettyPhoto[gallery]/1/

Kylie Minogue: I've NEVER had cosmetic surgery and I'm giving up Botox!
http://www.dailymail.co.uk/tvshowbiz/article-1280603/Kylie-Minogue-Ive-cosmetic-surgery-Im-giving-Botox.html#ixzz1srodnhhj
Yeah, as if!

Worse still is the media obsession with anyone who uses BOTOX®. Apparently, Simon Cowell has revealed in his new autobiography that he gets regular injections every four months (that's why he looks chubby faced). This information matters not to me, but he is an icon to the young and who (he knows better than most) have highly absorbent minds. In effect, he is saying yes to BOTOX®. Young minds are pliable and (do not reason that he is in his fifties). They only hear, that in order to be as successful as him use BOTOX®. I am not exaggerating and although I believe it was done innocently, moreover in good faith by him (in an attempt to be honest with his readership); I do feel that he should know better as he has made a fortune by fulfilling the "hopes and dreams" of the young people, their audiences and their peers.

I have tried in vain to start a campaign "Ban BOTOX® for Babes" to try to make it illegal for a mother to inject her child with BOTOX®, unfortunately no one was interested. In the USA Bill A3838 is going through the Senate.
http://www.njleg.state.nj.us/2010/Bills/A4000/3838_I1.HTM
Real celebrities were generally made famous by the profession they were in, be it in sports or entertainment. Because they are publicly recognisable personalities that various companies want to buy their services to promote their brands. By associating a celebrity with a product, the hope is that the brand will be thought

of alongside the press/media attention the celebrity normally receives automatically from their fame and also the celebrities' fans will naturally gravitate towards/or buy the product endorsed.

Celebrities are paid vast sums of money to endorse a product or products. The benefits to the celebrity are that in time, (especially lean times) the brand associated with the celebrity will stimulate interest in the celebrity. It is a win, win situation for the brand and the celebrity. The only losers in the situation are the public. I too am sucked in and like/wish to be associated with ABC celebrity and XYZ brand, so please do not misinterpret my words, I am merely stating business reality. The celebrities of today have business managers scouting out the best deals for their clients. Only today I read Jessie J was in debt before endorsing Domino's Pizza, MasterCard and Vitamin Water. Stars of yesteryear were no different; I recently heard on a TV documentary that Elizabeth Taylor made more money out of her perfume "White Diamonds" than she did from her film career

On the other hand, supermodels become famous either because - what they advertise sells well or because of the name brand they advertise was already famous. Models earn an honest living; they are paid to sell a product.

I am not knocking either and enjoy looking at the adverts for what they are – fantasy. Mutual cooperation for mutual long-term gain and profit; business! It is what it is, and makes the world go around. However, I do get frustrated by total and utter contempt of some of the complete advertising lies: that are allowed to be presented to an ever younger more receptacle, susceptible and possibly a more gullible audience. For example: advertising a hair conditioner, when the celebrity is wearing hair extensions – please! (Yes, in the small print they may now be forced to mention the fact but, in turning the magazine pages with fabulous Adobe® Photoshop® images and catchy captions; the small print is completely lost)!

Ultimately, I am sad to report that almost all the celebrity endorsements are unreal - in some shape, way or form. They are ONLY designed to sell products, and ONLY created to produce a desire in us to be transformed into a need, for us to purchase that particular product. Clever stuff, perhaps I should spend my time writing copy instead of the truth?

Unfortunately, if one does pick up a "fashion magazine" which shows all the latest fabulous and trends to inspire us, it is soon, most apparent, that they are almost entirely full of advertisement. Although one feels brighter initially, regrettably (having thumbed through the pages), one is left with the feeling of being lacking in some way, be it out of fashion, old and or ugly regardless of wardrobe, body weight and size or age, your face or just your look – don't fit. I do know this feeling from my past experiences of once being young, beautiful and having plenty of money; a wow. At that time, I could and did buy everything. I wanted (fabulous French face creams, designer clothes, fast cars and "whatever" money could buy) but still, I felt inadequate despite numerous compliments to the contrary!

Celebrity images

Today's celebrity's images are manufactured. The bigger they become the greater the illusion. The superstar's publicity agents try to control what is seen and read by the public.

For you to feel better about yourself and the reality of life, I strongly suggest that you cut out those moments when the celebrity is caught on camera in the local super market 'sans' makeup and not posing for the big event and place it side by side with a photograph of yourself looking at your best! **That is reality** as displayed when Felicity Kendal took a 'cigi' (cigarette) break in Strictly Come Dancing (U.K version) – ghastly despite all the work she has had done to her face! (More later, read on).

If you prefer, choose a photograph of the celebrity at his or her best, together with your collection of "their other photographs". Those that show reality, the star without makeup and each artificial procedures and interventions they have had (and will continuously have to) endure to maintain the false image generated.
At the end of the day, the big celebrities who are prepared to be steadfast in their endeavour to remain youthful still cannot beat the aging process. I do not think it's worth it, the constant battle against the clock. The other issue is that these celebrities are

beginning to look the same, without the individualism that made them famous in one way or another.

Ageless? It's so ageing Darling
I used to envy the Women Who Did It, but now, we're the ones having the last laugh. And to hell with the laughter lines
http://www.dailymail.co.uk/home/you/article-2111494/Ageless-It-s-ageing-darling.html#ixzz1qVDt7ksy

Adverts – photographs

With today's technologies, you can no longer believe what you see. It is no longer true that "A picture is worth a thousand words." Most, if not all, celebrity photographs are edited with Adobe® Photoshop®. The celebrities **have to** maintain their image and persona. Remember, celebrities are just people who became famous (to one degree or another) trying to make a living (in an ever increasingly competitive world). They too need to have the "edge." It is their business to 'look good', and it is the job of their entourage that includes many professionals to do if for them be it hair, makeup, stylists and their publicist. Their income depends entirely of their success of making their celebrity client look good. The celebrity's image is an advertisement to the world - which in many cases makes the product they are promoting. Subsequently, the product sells a million times more, that's why they are paid millions to look like a "million dollars." If not, they are dropped; it is as simple as that!
en.wikipedia.org/wiki/A_picture_is_worth_a_thousand_words

Photoshop (can and does make anyone look wonderful)
http://en.wikipedia.org/wiki/Adobe_Photoshop
Model sues over them not using Photoshop
http://www.beautyhigh.com/skin-caremodel-is-suing-over-not-being-photoshopped-in-ad/

Celebrity interviews, articles, half-truths and misinformation

It is any celebrities' business to 'look good'. In many cases, it is their primary focus of making a living, an income! Therefore, perhaps it is understandable that some of the older celebrities STILL REFUSE to admit to having had "work done;" from the knife or needles when it is blatantly obvious, for the entire world to see that something is amiss – but, still they pretend!

Why on earth do such people as Felicity Kendal keep pretending? When I saw her on Strictly Come Dancing I said to my mother "you see that twitch, that unconscious pouting of the lips, the pulled grimace, that's just like what Connie had in the States after her facelift – I told you, now you can see what I mean for yourself" Yet, Felicity Kendal totally denies it! Why? We the public (from the internet) even know the names of both her facelift surgeon and her BOTOX® doctor! I cannot comprehend why she has to say such blatant lies, it is lunacy. I can only empathise with her and think that perhaps she is mentally ill? I do not think that there is a person in the world who would stop liking her if she publicly stated that she had been lying and had had a facelift but was unable to face up to the fact herself.

Perhaps I am wrong and she is being responsible, not promoting intervention with surgery/fillers or too ashamed to admit that something went wrong judging from the appalling photo of her in the link below.

Felicity Kendal's eternally young life
http://www.dailymail.co.uk/tvshowbiz/article-404743/Felicity-Kendals-eternally-young-life.html

'Mr Botox' accused of negligence
http://www.dailymail.co.uk/news/article-1199932/Mr-Botox-accused-negligence.html

Eternal youth – in monthly doses
http://www.telegraph.co.uk/news/uknews/2021888/Eternal-youth-in-monthly-doses.html

Felicity is certainly not alone here in the UK in public denial of surgery or unnatural intervention with her face. Carol Vorderman is on the same plane. For those of you who may not know her she was made famous for being the "maths lady" on British TV show Countdown. Vorderman studied engineering at university, graduating with a third class degree. She is currently a presenter on Loose Women the UK equivalent of The View. Unbelievably only now at 52 has she declared that she may consider surgery in the future! PLEASE! She is so full of Botox and fillers that she is barely recognizable to the Countdown girl so good at maths.
http://en.wikipedia.org/wiki/Carol_Vorderman

'I'd look much better if I had been under the knife': Carol Vorderman insists she's never had surgery
http://www.dailymail.co.uk/tvshowbiz/article-2113389/Carol-Vordeman-insists-shes-surgery.html#ixzz1t3TCG4xb

It is not only the celebrities who lie but also some interviewers play along with the game and actually ask, "How do you continue to look so good" and the celebrity talks about nutrition and blushes!!! PLEASE. The public seems to be dazed - dazzled out of all sense of reality and forgets the recent photograph showing their idol with their face bandaged, coming out of a hospital post a facelift or coming out of rehab, for cocaine addiction!

The media too play the game with grabbing headlines like this one
50 WOMEN OVER 50 WHO HAVE AGED GRACEFULLY
The article talks all about aging gracefully, which I agree with. However with Madonna at Number 3, I didn't bother to read the article. It is the same whenever they introduce a mature celebrity and say, "How do you look so young?" as if we don't already know!
http://www.stylelist.com/2011/12/19/beautiful-women-over-50_n_1154571.html#s556474&title=Madonna_53

I should say, "the mind boggles" but I too am fooled, for a time!!

Once again, I stress the importance of thinking logically about reality. And if necessary to keep yourself in check with reality to keep a secret file of those shockingly true pictures of celebrities to remind yourself; that when you look in the mirror (first thing in the morning) that you are not so different after all!!
Celebrities Who Had The Worst Luck In Cosmetic Surgery
http://itthing.com/celebrity-cosmetic-surgery-fails

Celebrities all look alike

Whatever happened to individualism, to you being you? I can understand governments needing people to be sheep - to follow, there would be chaos otherwise; but please, when it comes to your individual identity and means to communicate effectively I urge you on the side of caution. Be yourself and REMEMBER that all the celebrities have had something done to themselves. Plus ALL the images have been through Photoshop before the celebrity's publicist even allowed them to be seen, on or in XYZ/magazine/newspaper/website. Only occasionally is an independent company brave enough to flout the rules – hence the "unseen" photographs – unbelievably even those can be and are (in some cases manipulated) to manipulate you!

Beautiful women over 50 - 50 sexiest women over 50
http://www.zimbio.com/The+50+Sexiest+Women+Over+50

The mirror and your perception of you

For goodness sake, give yourself a break and stop being so hard on yourself. Take a good hard long look in the mirror and like yourself! Be - happy that (at the very least) see your own image. What is the famous expression? "A blind man would be glad to see you" YES – remember that. He would be thrilled and delighted to see your image; be you short, tall, fat or seriously ugly - it would make that previously blind person ecstatically happy beyond belief. There will always be someone more beautiful - or richer, or cleverer, or taller or kinder or better than you.

Stop illogically competing with unreality.

If you are very young (to me, in your twenties or under) and your Mum showed you this page in my book (because you too were feeling as insure - as I did at your age), you would probably think to yourself, "What does she know?"

Well, probably quite a lot! She may tell you that those very people, who are trying to put you down, are, in reality, probably jealous of you. Or she may be trying to give you inspiration or inner courage. This world has six (or is it now closer to 7 billion people living on the planet and not everyone will think you are attractive – it really doesn't matter, only to you.

Although I do facial exercise, and write about them, my looks or rather (as I age) the lack of them means that, in reality, I am a HAS BEEN and was only a "10" for a brief period of my life. Fortunately, I relatively easily come to terms with it. Age is age, which does bring its consolations. Good looks are SO OVERATED. I had them, naturally for a while, and I was bloody miserable for the duration of my twenties!

However, I would be the first to agree that they good looks open doors, that if for no one else they seem to matter to oneself, to me in my fifties. Therefore, my only advice is that if you are still youngish, in your thirties, or forties, I strongly suggest that you do not waste any more time and try the exercises in this book – you have nothing to lose.

If you are adaptable, sensible and perhaps in your fifties - you probably think and feel that perhaps you have left it a bit too late to do anything; well yes and no. My oldest person to first try to do facial exercises was a man of 72 (he bought a book), but I did not make contact so cannot claim to verify any positive results. A good girlfriend of mine tried them, in earnest, at 51 years of age and said "she could not continue because her face hurt!" With all the other pressures that she had to contend with in life she gave up! Pity, she had her priorities. My point being is that at whatever age you begin face exercises they work. However, (like most things in life), it does all depend on you and your commitment plus how far you have let yourself go. Even like an honest cosmetic surgeon, (of which, I am sure there are many) I cannot promise to make you look wonderful, but exercise is the best natural way forward to rejuvenate your face and give you a healthy natural glow for a lifetime.

I am now beginning to feel sorry for the older celebrities who have become victims of plastic surgery, forever repairing the damage done when they were younger. Yes, I can understand when one is young wanting to look fabulous, just like the latest celebrity. But before you start messing up your face with damaging unnatural intervention take a long hard look at these idols. Some do look good NOW, but I ask you, "Will they be as attractive in their 60s or 70s as someone who has only had minor work done later in life?
I doubt it; there is a heavy price to pay later in life for too early intervention with needles and knives. Many just give up, accept reality and get off of the painful merry-go-round such as Hilary Clinton.

Surgery Celebs (PHOTOS)
http://www.huffingtonpost.co.uk/2012/04/15/surgery-celebs-photos_n_1426745.html?icid=maing-grid7%7Cuk%7Cdl7%7Csec1_lnk3%26pLid%3D105158
Plastic Surgery: Keeping Celebrities Looking Old and Stupid

http://www.cagle.com/2012/03/plastic-surgery-keeping-celebrities-looking-old-and-stupid/

Even some young stars regret Botox and surgery, like Jordan and Hedi Montag.
Heidi Montag reveals her scars a year after surgery
http://www.lifeandstylemag.com/2010/12/heidi-cover-story.html

Needles and knives do ultimately lead to some very sad, deformed, irregular, unnatural, damaged faces. Face exercises do not. So who REALLY wants to end up looking like them anyway?

I, together with some other enlightened woman, all over the planet are trying to put the idea of 'health before beauty' and that euphoric feeling of self-esteem back into the lives of young people. Unfortunately in today's world many youngsters feel 'lacking' in some shape, way or form. I grew up feeling VERY, VERY UNHAPPY because I believed (and up to a point it was true) that I was really fat. I can still hear the humiliating chants and jeers shouted by my angelic looking classmates on Sports Day at our private school (a convent) as I pathetically tried to run (with my wobbly thighs rubbing together) towards the finish line in the egg and spoon race. Needless to say I was always last by a mile. The team that drew me, in whatever sport, drew the short straw!

If you feel strongly about any of the issues raised in this book do look on the internet (regardless of your age or country) there you may find a group that you can associate with and support. Personally, I have chosen **Body Confidence** (the co-founder of which is a beautiful young British member of parliament) and to a much lesser extent I empathise with **AnyBody** also here in the U.K. There are too many and too diverse in the USA to list here.
Body confidence and the new political line on beauty
http://www.guardian.co.uk/commentisfree/2012/apr/20/body-confidence-new-line-on-beauty
campaignforbodyconfidence
http://campaignforbodyconfidence.wordpress.com/
Body confidence campaign
http://www.homeoffice.gov.uk/equalities/equality-government/body-confidence/
Body confidence awards

http://www.guardian.co.uk/fashion/2012/apr/20/body-confidence-awards-fightback

Chair person convenor and of Anybody
She is a psychotherapist, psychoanalyst, writer, and social critic
http://en.wikipedia.org/wiki/Susie_Orbach
http://www.any-body.org/

Chapter 2

Why we age
How to prevent premature aging

How to glow with healthy good looks
By doing facial exercises that work

Looking good - is all about the face and the skin - projecting a glowing, healthy, wrinkle and blemish free skin to the on looking world. How is this achieved and more importantly how is it maintained for a lifetime?

The key to staying or looking beautiful forever is **knowledge.** Knowledge is power. There is a vast array of information out there on the internet, freely available to all. But, some of it is misinformation at best, while most of it is propaganda used to influence fresh young minds to buy products in the hope of gaining a customer for a lifetime. In a way I am doing the same, although I have your best interests at heart and my advice over a lifetime is virtually free.

I may sound cynical to the young, but think of me like your mother - whom no doubt has told you, not to waste your money on this or that" because from her experience, (despite the claims) many products don't do what they say they can on the fancy package. She cares about you and doesn't want you to make the same mistakes as her, nevertheless we all do!

Maybe you are a mother yourself and have noticed the odd wrinkle or two appearing. Perhaps you have tried some skin care creams and been disappointed with the results. Now possibly you are considering something more invasive like the needle. Before you take that next very serious step please do read on, and learn how to maintain a youthful beautiful face forever. For once you start with injections it is a downward spiral of dependency, like creams that break promises so do injections. It all starts well enough with a Botox type injection but like with most addictive substances you will need more sooner, and then it's on to fillers. And after they fail and your face is all puffed up beyond recognition the only way left is the knife! The alternative is Fitface facial exercises, where you can remain looking wonderful for a lifetime.

If you are mature reader, my age is 56 (born in 1956), you may have been through many miracle creams and perhaps the odd injection or two; none of which have lasted and now perhaps, desperate you could be thinking of the dreaded knife. Please do stop, read on and learn. You cannot turn back the clock forever even with the knife. Facelifts do not last. Aging is natural.

Please stop kidding yourself. You are not a major international celebrity or your PA would be reading this book for you. Celebrity photo opportunities on mature ladies are just that, red carpet fully staged events. One can name such celebrities on one's hands. They spend every waking moment prior to the event "getting ready" from nutritionist preparing menus for their chefs to surgery and stems cell injections plus hormonal injections. Despite all the money spent, the pain endured, and what they have had to put themselves through for their careers/fame/fortunes, they still (without the right lightening/makeup/Adobe® Photoshop®) look like their age, (be it well preserved), which is what they are! Regrettably, some look freakish.

Enough of my observations, let's move on to the meat of the exercise. How to make you look wonderful forever - it's so simple:

Firstly, obtain the knowledge on what happens inside your face and body to make the difference on the outside.

Secondly, act on that information. In the short term that is easy. We all get motivated to do something for a short while with encouragement, but keeping it up is something different. Even I have problems keeping motivated.

I hope that by the time you read this I have established some sort of webcam connection with my readers so that when they are down or need some advice or encouragement they can reach me via Skype.

Natural facial aging phenomena

We all age and (as yet) there is nothing we can do to stop it.

Mother Nature favours the survival of the fittest for reproduction and proliferation of the species. The weak and old are redundant, by-products from the main objective.

Our attraction to beauty (or rather to locate a healthy 'mate' for reproduction purposes) is hard wired into our DNA over millions and millions of years. Our obsession with a youthful, glowing physical appearance is only natural. It is the natural order.

Communication

We are the most successful predator on the planet. Why? We are not the biggest or the strongest. It is because we learned to communicate with each other. We formed groups, socialised and hunted together and as they say, "the rest is history."

In short, our ability to communicate made us the top predator. This developed from facial expressions into language - yet 92% of all communication is body language. I wonder how much of communication is facial?. I feel a Google moment coming on.

A facial expression is one or more motions or positions of the muscles in the skin. These movements convey the emotional state of the individual to observers. Facial expressions are a form of nonverbal communication. They are a primary means of conveying social information among humans, and also occur in most other mammals and some other animal species.
http://en.wikipedia.org/wiki/Facial_expression

Non-verbal communication remains the earliest form of communication beginning with our mothers and others through facial expression. The face was and is the focus of our primary attention.
http://en.wikipedia.org/wiki/Nonverbal_communication

Professor Albert Mehrabian has pioneered the understanding of communications since the 1960's. He received his Ph.D. from Clark University and in 1964 commenced an extended career of teaching and research at the University of California, Los Angeles. He currently devotes his time to research, writing, and consulting as Professor Emeritus of Psychology, UCLA. Aside from his many and various other fascinating works, Mehrabian established this classic statistic for the effectiveness of spoken communications:
- 7% of meaning is in the words that are spoken.
- 38% of meaning is paralinguistic (the way that the words are said).
- 55% of meaning is in facial expression.

http://jefmenguin.wordpress.com/resources/articles/professor-albert-mehrabians-communications-model/

We have developed as a species that loves to communicate. Yes, paradoxically with all the sophisticated ways to communicate that are available to communicate we actually communicate less face-to-face. This is a worrying trend! The history, the character and the very essence of a person is etched on the face. Over millions of years we have learned (for our survival) to recognize even the most obscure, minute difference in facial expression to alert us of danger. In today's language, a look, just an eye movement can let us know that this person – despite what they are saying, our instinct/brain tells us they are not all they are cracked up to be. We read facial expressions subconsciously a little like a lie detector test and rarely are our inherent instincts incorrect.

How many times have you seen "the look" good or bad and you know exactly what it means. Be it from a besotted lover, a glance of admiration, a filthy look from a so called friend, the look of envy, anger or just plain hatred. I think I have made my point.

Facial expression

Without being too dramatic or deep, teaching our young survival skills is essential for the survival of the species. Our ancestor's ability to communicate was the key to our success. Therefore, for me, it is sad to watch our newly born infant babies try to communicate with their mothers who have had BOTOX® type injections. All the natural nuances of facial expression i.e. communications are lost.

It is sad to think that we have come so far, yet learned nothing! Even I remember the experiments with monkeys dating back about 25 years ago whereby a monkey would choose to hug a fur covered robot rather than be fed with milk by a non-fur covered robot, such is our DNA. To go against Mother Nature is to go against the grain, which ultimately will incur her wrath.

Young mothers who use BOTOX® type injections cannot communicate effectively with their babies. There are many examples on YouTube, but I cannot bring myself to publish the links to them as they are too distressing.

My message is simple:
Yes, "Beauty" matters."
Yes, "Staying youthful-looking" matters.
So together; let's do something about it NATURALLY.

Skipping the details

Please by all means feel free to miss chunks of this book; much is the science behind why facial exercises work. If you already know or are convinced, just skip on.

Why the face ages first

The face appears to age more readily than the rest of us, again this is natural. Our faces are exposed to the elements; therefore its effects of our lives are revealed to the world, or rather as nature intended to any "would-be" mate.

Our head contains our brains and all our five sense organs for sight, hearing, taste, smell and touch (all over your body) as your face, lips and neck are some of the most sensitive parts to touch.

Once again, Mother Nature; put all the essential things in one place which was in order to make you and your lifestyle publicly on display to strangers to potential mates. The face shows off your condition - your age – which designed by nature shows off your ability or not to produce healthy offspring!

Visible signs of facial aging
- Wrinkles
- Folds
- Crepe like skin
- Sagging face
- Sunken cheeks
- Age spots
- Dry skin
- Hair loss
- Grey hair
- Eyelash thinning and shortening
- Dull eyes
- Facial hairs
- Shrunken head
- Double chin
- Colourless skin
- Thinning skin
- Melasma (chloasma) an unspoken possible side effect of HRT. (I developed this which has now disappeared as I stopped taking HRT)
  http://en.wikipedia.org/wiki/Melasma

Reasons for aging

The most fundamental overriding reason for facial aging, even in today's world is the natural aging process. Our face and body are made up of cells; which age over time and the body tissues degenerate. It is a highly complex process that is constantly being researched and different basic theories have emerged. But thus far **NO ONE HAS EVER ESCAPED AGING OR DYING.** They are now trying with senescent cells:

http://www.bbc.co.uk/news/health-15552964

The underlying, causes of natural aging

Loss of bone density
Loss of facial fat pads
Loss of elastin (elasticity)
Loss of skin tone (complex degeneration)
Loss of collagen
Loss of muscle tone from muscle wastage
Loss of hormone production

Intrinsic and Extrinsic Aging

Basically (allowing for DNA/genetics – studies on twins) both are under our control but only up to a point.

Intrinsic aging - Internal factors

The effects of intrinsic aging are caused primarily by internal factors alone. It is sometimes referred to as chronological aging and is an inherent degenerative process due to declining physiologic functions and capacities. Such an aging process may include qualitative and quantitative changes and includes diminished or defective synthesis of collagen and elastin in the dermis.

Extrinsic aging - External factors

Extrinsic aging of skin is a distinctive declination process caused by external factors which include ultra-violet radiation, cigarette smoking and air pollution, among many other things. Of all extrinsic causes, radiation from sunlight has the most widespread documentation of its negative effects on the skin:
http://en.wikipedia.org/wiki/Intrinsic_and_extrinsic_aging

Perhaps in time they will add surgery, fillers and Botox type injections to the list of factors that cause extrinsic aging? It is not only me, I am not alone. If you do your homework and can get past the array of advertising and editorials, you'll find many articles on the internet which suggest the same.

How to have a healthy glowing skin

My best advice (which will do absolutely nothing for sales of this book) would be for you to go to a desert island alone or with a lover and do absolutely nothing about skincare or facial exercise! On the rare occasions in life that I have done just that, let go of the way I looked and just felt lucky to be alive my face responded positively too. Was it because nature had been allowed to kick in?

I gave my experiences some more analysis and thought; why am I so surprised? In nature; do you see dirty animals? No! Never; well not often in nature, only the sick, old or near dying. It is very rare to see an unkempt animal; if you do they are normally sick. Most animals have glossy silk coats and svelte, trim, toned bodies. They are not over toxically fed, obese, media affected, avid mass consumers. Unfortunately even some animals have fallen prey to their owner's obsession with modern consumerism and become unnatural pampered pouches.

What was the answer? To do nothing in today's unforgiving consumer orientated world? No; of course not. Within a week of returning from one of my escapades I was back to normal, back in the hub of consumerism and if not "loving it" certainly towing the line.

So what is the answer?

Change your mindset

Treat the face as an extension of the body. It is not a separate unit. All the things that you would do to make your body work better apply to the face. The fitness guru Jack LaLanne who won many, many awards and lived until he was 96 incorporated the face into his exercise routines.

Think and act young, youthful, in love with life - to look like it. That much is obvious, but we need to be consciously doing it.

The natural aging process and personal genetics are responsible for some of the affects of the visible signs of aging. There are a host of other things that can be done to prevent premature aging and even reverse the clock both naturally and artificially. (I will discuss more radical intervention later).

All that is needed to either begin or remain looking lovely, with glowing healthy skin is a commitment to a change in your lifestyle habits. Prevention is far better than a cure and the most important thing you can do is start where you mean to end.

- **Start young**

As with most positive things you do in life, the earlier you start the better. Practice makes perfect, one becomes totally established in a routine over time and things become second nature to you. We all know that the opposite is true; sadly bad habits are very hard to break.

The basic problem is that we don't listen, especially when we are young. We don't listen, we don't want to listen (let alone understand) to our mothers' who were almost always right, and we certainly don't/won't listen to our grandmothers! "As if they know anything at their age, get real!"

I didn't listen to my mother telling me to "stop wasting your money" on this or that fantastic new cosmetic product - in those days it was a conditioner. In today's world I attempt to do the same and try to tell my daughter that claims made by a celebrity maybe untrue and that they earned serious money for, saying "it worked." Worse; nowadays models/celebrities can get away with murder, for example; they can wear hair extensions and advertise a shampoo! I just thought about my mother, who was and still is a grumpy old woman – now I'm saying the same! When she was reading through my first draft of this book she commented on this section and said, "Charlotte, that was Cheryl Cole - I think you ought to mention it!" So I am, I went on to tell her that in today's world false advertising is okay so long as you add the "disclaimer" i.e. tell the reader/world in small print that the model (in that example) is wearing hair extensions, false eyelashes or whatever. My mother listened perplexed, dazed by the reality of the changing world in which she now lives. She knows I speak the truth and like me is astonished.

Yes, when much younger I did try every lotion and potion and cream on the market – none did anything and some brought me out in a rash!

Interestingly my mother can raise each eyebrow independently which I cannot *and believe me I have tried.* She told me that as a little girl she was infatuated by the way that the American GI's would wink - with one eyebrow raised - at her older sister. (During the 2nd World War she was between 9 and 14 and her older sister between 14 & 19 years old). So, at home my mother practiced the movement to be "cool." She is now 81 and although she hardly ever does it, she can still perform this party trick. When she shows me, she also often recants that her mother (my grandmother) used to wear a piece of Elastoplast (Band-Aid) between her eyebrows to prevent her frowning – an interesting early BOTOX®! The message is that muscles do learn.

- **Combat nature with nature**

For me and the scientific community it stands to reason that if nature makes you age then nature must be challenged to slow down the processes. We grow from the inside out, what we put in our bodies (nourishment/hydration) and how we burn what we eat (exercise) expel waste products, and how we feel will show on our faces. This is what nature intended for us, to be able to recognise a healthy mate in order to reproduce and propagate the species!

- **Don't do anything unnatural**

Drugs, excessive drinking of alcohol, and smoking cigarettes significantly decrease the supply of oxygen to skin cells. Staying in bed all day because you are depressed is not good for the skin. Get out and get some exercise, get some exposure to natural sunlight or fresh air, you will feel better and therefore, look better.

Basically doing or not doing anything that your body was not designed for is detrimental to your physical or mental health it affects your skin – be it too much partying or stress at work.

Injecting Botox is not natural. The Journal of Cosmetic Dermatology in 2002, Dr David Becker, an assistant professor of dermatology at Weill Cornell Medical College in New York, observed that "wrinkles caused by untreated muscles of facial expression paradoxically can become more prominent."

"Paralysis of a set of muscles," he suggests, "might lead to recruitment of other muscle groups in an attempt to reproduce the conditioned activity being blocked - resulting in more prominent muscle activity in adjacent regions."

In other words, your face will still find a way to make expressions by using different facial muscles where you've had not had BOTOX® injected into the muscle, which therefore leads to more lines.
http://www.dailymail.co.uk/femail/beauty/article-1275841/Botox-backlash-Evidence-reveals-called-miracle-jab-actually-GIVE-wrinkles.html#ixzz1srQBRALr

- **Eat nourishing food**

Skin grows from the inside out. It does matter what you eat. Your face and body need good nutrition – best found in real wholesome unprocessed foods. Sadly, even if you try to eat the finest fresh fruit and vegetables daily, the soil in which commercial crops are grown has lost much of its nutritional value. Hence those essential minerals, salts and vitamins are not transferred to the food we eat today.

My advice would be to eat organically grown food produced locally in season. That's all well and good but I don't. However, I do go to farmers' markets, support "grown in Britain," and at least try not to overcook the vitamins out of fresh foods and (100% fail to) cut out all processed foods! What is the expression? *"Do as I say, not do as I do!*

I like much of the information in The World Healthiest Foods by George Mateljan, sold in the USA via Wholefoods.
http://www.whfoods.com/newbook/bookannounce.html
Nutrition
http://en.wikipedia.org/wiki/Nutrition
What to Eat for Glowing Healthy Skin
www.sciencedaily.com/releases/2007/11/071109201438.htm
Nourishing your skin. Great diet great skin

http://www.webmd.com/healthy-aging/features/nourishing-your-skin

One of the worst things in processed foods is salt

- **Limit sugar intake**

Sugar is the number-one collagen destroyer, especially alcohol, (she writes as she sips a cool glass of Sauvignon Blanc).

Glycation: is a body process that involves the attachment of sugars (travelling in the bloodstream) to proteins, which produce a molecule that damages the collagen and elastin in the skin. In short - the more sugar you eat, the more collagen and elastin killer molecules are produced by your body. Once these fibres are damaged, they become dry and brittle, which ultimately will lead to wrinkles and sagging of the facial skin.
http://ezinearticles.com/?Foods-That-Cause-Wrinkles&id=6892363
Face Facts: Too much sugar can cause wrinkles
http://www.nutrition-info.com/nutrientdestroyers.php
Nutrient destroyers
http://www.nutrition-info.com/nutrientdestroyers.php
The sweet truth: Ditch sugar to look ten years younger
http://www.dailymail.co.uk/femail/article-461095/The-sweet-truth-Ditch-sugar-look-years-younger.html#ixzz1r4YuicPo
'High Doses Of Sugar Is The Same As Poison' Warns Doctor Robert Lustig' A paediatric endocrinologist from the University of California
http://www.huffingtonpost.co.uk/2012/04/03/high-doses-sugar-toxic-poison_n_1399038.html?

- **Drink plenty of water**

Skin is hydrated from the inside out. It does matter what you drink. Your face and body needs hydration – best found in water.

Water – The Essential Nutrient
http://www.internethealthlibrary.com/Environmental-Health/WaterTheEssentialNutrient.htm
Drinking Water to Improve Your Complexion
http://skin-care-facial-care.factoidz.com/drinking-water-to-improve-your-complexion/

Drink More Water for Beautiful Skin
http://www.beautifulskinblog.com/2007/11/drink-more-water-to-get-healthy-skin.html
http://www.celebrity-beauty-tip-goldmine.com/great-skin.html

Personally I think tap water is as healthy, if not better than bottled water, only because bottled water is "manufactured." It has been transported from the source, filtered, processed, stored, shipped and stored on the shelf. During this time, the temperature of the original product has been changed and in hot climates, the plastic bottles are likely to have been exposed to extensive sunlight and then refrigerated. Therefore, I ask myself, "What can be left of the original product when one unscrews the bottle cap?"

- **Limit your exposure to the elements**

Protect the delicate facial skin with a protective barrier from excessive exposure to sunlight, the wind and cold. But do let your face breathe; go outside - don't stay in the air conditioning or central heating those actions are unhealthy - skin killers too.

Harsh weather conditions
Enduring extreme temperatures and winds without adequate moisturisers and protection prematurely ages the skin

UV radiation
Likewise, neglecting to protect the skin from the sun's UV rays with sunscreen ages the facial skin

Wrinkles are the result of collagen breakdown in the dermis. Sunlight destructs collagen fibres in the skin, which provokes the build up of abnormal elastin and the metalloproteinase enzymes, are accumulated in abundance. When the normal metalloproteinase enzymes are in charge of the remodelling of the sun-damaged skin they remake the lost collagen.
http://en.wikipedia.org/wiki/Metalloproteinase

When the process is not accurately carried out, these enzymes break the collagen down. The result is the arrangement of disordered collagen fibres that are formerly known as 'solar scars'. As time goes by, and these solar scars are repeatedly damaged

by the sun and as long as this imperfect process is persistent then wrinkles will be formed (worsening as more time goes by).
http://www.healthyskincream.com/sundamage/

- **Reduce stress**

We have all heard that stress is the number one killer, well not only does it harm the body, it also harms the skin. Stress causes wrinkles and ages the skin. It does matter what you think and feel. Stress will show on your face, not only with tension (at the time) that will cause dynamic wrinkles but also permanently unless you do facial exercises to relax and smooth away tight muscle tension.

What Are the Effects of Cortisol and How Does It Affect My Health?
http://www.holistic-mindbody-healing.com/effects-of-cortisol.html
Effects of Stress on Your skin
http://www.webmd.com/healthy-beauty/guide/the-effects-of-stress-on-your-skin

Negative Effects of Cortisol
Stress studies done on rats, show that collagen loss in the skin was ten times greater than in any other tissue. Remember that during stress the body prioritizes what is important for "fight or flight." Wrinkle-free, young-looking skin is not one of those priorities.
http://www.holistic-mindbody-healing.com/effects-of-cortisol.html
Cortisol and Stress:
http://stress.about.com/od/stresshealth/a/cortisol.htm

- **Keep up with your age, including skin care regime**

Be it clothes, hair or makeup – information and products change. Go with the flow and keep up with the current pace, tends and innovations. Not only will you look more 'with it' you will feel brighter as well.

Skin care changes too as you age naturally and grow older. As you age the sloughing off of dead cells from the surface of your skin will change. Pre, during and after menopause you will need to exfoliate more often, which is unnecessary in your youth (leave it to nature). With age dead skin does not shed at the same rate;

that is not to say that I recommend chemical peels I DO NOT. They are far too abrasive, especially for thinning delicate tissues. *Why would you inflict further damage on damaged skin?*

Exfoliation is a technique whereby the layer of dead epidermal cells on the outer surface of the skin (a.k.a. stratum corneum) is removed to expose fresher mostly living cells. Potential benefits of exfoliation include fresher, brighter looking skin, better penetration of active ingredients of skin-care products and, for people with excessively oily skin, a varying degree of reduction in oil secretion.
http://www.smartskincare.com/skincarebasics/basicexfoliation.html

A dull, rough complexion is another visible sign of skin aging. Healthy, young skin remains smooth and radiant because fresh, new cells are brought up to the surface as older cells are continuously shed. The skin cells in the bottom layer of the epidermis (stratum basale) constantly divide through cell division, forming new keratinocytes. This regenerative process is called skin cell renewal. As we age, the rate of skin cell renewal decreases, causing cells to become stickier and not shed as easily. As a result of cell renewal decreasing, the skin becomes thinner and more susceptible to environmental damage, especially photo damage from the sun's UV rays. Eventually, the skin appears dull and rough in texture.
http://www.nuskin.com/en_ZA/corporate/company/science/skin_care_science/skin_aging_and_physiology.html

- **Exercise**

We all know that exercise is good for you. Why? It improves your health by lowering blood pressure, improving circulation and cholesterol. Some of the other major benefits of exercise are:

- Controls weight
- Stimulates growth hormones
- Builds muscles either to promote endurance and/or strength
- Builds collagen
- Improves mood
- Improves memory

- Reduces stress
- Speeds up our reaction times
- Improves balance
- Increases our flexibility
- Increases bone strength and protects against fractures
- Improves our psychological health
- Improves sleep
- Improves sex life

http://www.mayoclinic.com/health/exercise/HQ01676
http://lifelearningtoday.com/2008/04/18/why-is-exercise-good-for-you/
http://www.dumblittleman.com/2008/02/13-scientifically-proven-health.html

Aging & What You Can Do About It
There is a large body of scientific evidence that suggests that we can slow down and even reverse the symptoms of aging. In fact many of us can be in better health in our 70's than we were in our 50's.
http://www.befitoverfifty.com/
Exercises for Good Health At Any Age
http://ladytrainerstogo.com/personal-trainer-articles/exercise-for-good-health.htm
It's never too late to start exercising
http://abclocal.go.com/wabc/story?section=news/health&id=8539384

- **Face exercise**

The face is covered with facial muscles to form expression, and the whole face and neck is attached to muscular fibre extending from the forehead to the back of the neck. To keep the face toned and in shape, exercise is required; just as the body needs exercising.

Face exercise for your five sense organs

For me, it is just common sense. Surely, it stands to reason that if regular exercise is that good for keeping the body toned and in tune then surely the same applies to the head?

Furthermore, in fact, would it not be fair to say that the head is the most important part of the body? Is that not the only region of the body, where all of our five senses can be found?

The sense organs, senses are
- hearing
- sight
- touch
- smell
- taste

http://en.wikipedia.org/wiki/Five_senses
http://en.wikipedia.org/wiki/Sense

Would it not also be fair to say that the functionality of your senses/sense organs is of primary importance to the quality of your life? Are not all these senses in your head? Therefore, surely it makes sense to ensure an adequate supply of fresh oxygenated blood from exercise would be good for the five sense organs?

Good health is about the whole body and face, taking responsibility for your life and how you age. It is not all about the way you look. To look good you must feel good and part of that is your general health.

Moreover, and most importantly your head contains your brain which you cannot live without! I will not write about it here, only plant the idea as food for thought. We all know that we can only live 4 minutes without oxygen delivered by the blood. You can explore more about what aging and an oxygen depleted blood supply does to the brain at the link below.
http://en.wikipedia.org/wiki/Vertebrobasilar_insufficiency

Why facial exercises are good for you

Facial exercises are a great way to get healthy radiant looking skin regardless of your age. Yes, exercises are anti-aging too. Face exercises are a fantastic natural method to prevent premature aging without the expense and/or risks of plastic surgery or injections.

Many people say that doing facial exercises has tightened and firmed up sagging and loose skin. Unfortunately there are only a few studies on the subject that exist. Without exercise, the muscles in any part of the body become flaccid and atrophy. Exercising the face is a natural way to tone up the muscles and give the appearance that the skin has been lifted. Facial exercises let you improve the look of your skin from the inside out.

Why exercise the facial muscles?

The face moves because of the underlying muscles. For the most part the facial skin is attached to the muscles, and this makes it possible for facial expressions such as smiling, raising an eyebrow, frowning or winking. The skin and muscles of the face are closely connected.

As we age, the muscles and tissue fibres decrease and degrade, leaving drooping and lined skin, wrinkles and folds. The skin is attached to the subcutaneous tissue and the muscles. For the most part the muscles are interconnected with other muscles. As the facial muscles are contracted and relaxed, the muscles and tissue fibres increase in volume, (similar to body building) increasing the size of muscles. With stronger and tighter facial muscles, the underlying tissues are strengthened, and this affects the skin by reducing the appearance of wrinkles and loose skin.

After the muscles have been exercised the skin is gently plumped up naturally from underneath and fractionally stretched, which results in a smoother and more taut, toned face. The signs of aging are diminished. Facial exercise also increases the production of collagen.

Why do facial exercises?

To prevent premature aging and gain a great toned, fit face. Face exercises are a natural and inexpensive way to gain a more youthful toned appearance. Exercising the body is known to help tone up the muscles, to make them larger, stronger and more defined. The same applies to the face.

If you don't exercise the body, the body will lose tone. The same thing happens to the face and it worsens overtime. Exercising the facial muscles has the same effect as exercising the legs or abdomen. Facial exercise can not only prevent wrinkles, sagging skin and dropping eyelids, but it can also reverse some of the damage already done by aging. Facial exercises affect people differently. By simply doing facial exercises on a daily basis for 5 to 10 minutes, you can see an improvement within a few weeks. Facial exercises work by focusing on one set of facial muscles at a time to strengthen the entire surrounding facial muscles - not just one. Exercise also brings oxygen and nutrient-rich blood to the face, and these are important for the function and maintenance of skin cells.

Studies and Research

In a study conducted by Gary L. Grove, PhD, at the Skin Study Centre, a research facility in Pennsylvania, after 3 months of twice-daily facial exercises, the participants showed "highly significant differences." The participants felt their faces were more firm and more elastic. The facial muscles were also stronger "as measured by the time they could hold a high resistance load."
How Does Doing Facial Exercises Firm Face Muscles?
http://www.ehow.com/how-does_4657247_facial-exercises-firm-face-muscles.html#ixzz1rG3n32XN

How are facial wrinkles formed?

There are two types of wrinkle movements, **dynamic** and **static** wrinkles (more in the next chapter). We move the muscles in our faces to communicate a facial expression, for example, a frown which forms a dynamic wrinkling of the skin. With years and years of a repetitive action, the once dynamic only movements become static, (stationary, stuck). This happens because the muscle does not relax and unwind; it does not go back to its relaxed state but remains tensed up. The wrinkle literally gets "stuck in a groove." The muscle has learned to stay put, that muscle becomes dominate and the other muscles weaken because they are not being used. As this happens the collagen gets pushed aside and pulled down, flattened, diminished, and stiffened. Again the collagen is stuck, not unravelled or unwound but fixed. Both the muscle and collagen are stuck, pulling the skin down into the fold.
Most of the muscles within the body are attached at either end to bone. However, in the face they are not. Most muscles in the face

are attached at one end only to bone with tendinous fibre or ligaments, and the other end inserted into the skin. Whenever the skin is pulled down by a muscle contraction to form a facial movement or an expression, a crease is formed. Muscles learn and with repetitive movements over time the most moved muscle gains the most strength and the supporting surrounding muscles loose strength, hence exacerbating the depth and pull of that muscle. Without use, those other muscles weaken "muscular atrophy." (Something like when a victim of a car accident loses the use of his or her legs and they waste away).

Therefore, it makes perfect sense that to unfix, stop or prevent wrinkles from forming in the first place one must do facial exercises to strengthen ALL the facial muscles to prevent the onset of any one facial muscle from becoming dominant. Hence the expression "if you don't use it you'll lose it" when related to exercise.
Muscle atrophy - http://"en.wikipedia.org/wiki/Muscle_atrophy

I find it strange that BOTOX® (a neurotoxin prescription medicine that is injected into muscles) has become an unwitting friend to facial exercise advocates, since both methods produce the same end result – muscle relaxation. However, there are major differences in how each of the results is achieved, along with both the possible short and the long-term consequences.

With facial exercises, the results are achieved naturally. There are better long-term results because facial muscles do not work in isolation of each other. For the most part, facial muscles blend and inter-cross with one another and other muscles, therefore, when you tone one muscle, you tone many others and build the essential collagen too. They work together in natural harmony.

On the other hand, BOTOX® is artificial. Muscle relaxation can be achieved by an injection of the neurotoxin into a specific muscle. The toxin can reach other parts of the body and brain. BOTOX® can cause death and disfigurement and the consequences of long-term use are as yet unknown. All drugs with a **black box warning** carry a significant risk of severe and "life-threatening effects." **BOTOX® carries a black box warning**

BOTOX® blocks signals from the nerves to the muscles. The injected muscles can no longer contract, which causes the wrinkles to relax and soften for a time, until the next injection!
http://en.wikipedia.org/wiki/Botulinum_toxin

Because BOTOX® is generally only injected into one or two facial muscles, the other muscles are not strengthened, and collagen is not built up - unlike facial exercise, which does increase collagen. *For me it makes perfect common sense to include facial exercise in my exercise routine if for no other reason than to increase collagen.*

The long term-effects of BOTOX® are as yet unknown. It has only been around 20 years. However, we do know that it causes Wrinklerexia and addition to the point of deformity. Facial exercise has no negative side effects. JackLanne did facial exercises all his life and did not die until 96 and looked wonderful. *I think that speaks for itself, as to the positive long-term effects of facial exercises.*

Exercise increases collagen

In an excerpt I discovered posted online September 11, 2009 Yafa Sakkejha wrote, "Professor Stuart Warden, Director of Physical Therapy Research at Indiana University, informed the New York Times last week that "the stresses of exercise activate a particular molecular pathway that increases collagen," which leads to stronger connective tissues in the dermis, and thus, fewer wrinkles and younger-looking skin.

Collagen is essential; making up about 25% to 35% of the whole-body protein content.
http://en.wikipedia.org/wiki/Collagen

What can Fitface do for you?

Fitface will make you feel great
Because you have taken responsibility
not only for the way you look
but also the health of your face and sense organs.

Our face is the face that the world sees and
(like it or not) the world judges you by your face.
Put your best face forward and be all that you can be.
Give your face to the finest natural spa
Fitface - works for you from the inside out

Start today to see a more radiant, glowing, and healthier, looking you staring back at yourself in the mirror

Fitface is a non-invasive, beauty spa beauty treatment system Fitface is a facial workout used to stimulate the skin, plus all the muscles of the face, neck and décolletage naturally.

Used regularly Fitface maintains younger looks A fresher brighter face, skin and hair will dramatically reduce any further signs of aging

The results you will notice:

Glow – increased circulation hydrates your complexion
Facial contours - lifted
Frown lines - minimised
Crow's feet - softened
Brow furrows - lessened
Eyes - hoods lifted, bags diminished
Cheeks - plumped out, - re- shaped
Nasolabial folds - eased out
Lips - fuller
Jowls - lifted
Jaw line - more defined
Neck - toned
Double chin - reduced

Décolletage - increased tautness and hence less wrinkled

Fitface benefits are amazing – no women should be without it.

Top 10 reasons to do" hands free" facial exercises

- **Achieve a glowing healthy looking skin**
- **Build up collagen**
- **Prevent static wrinkles and skin folds**
- **Stimulate healthy thick hair growth**
- **Lift sags and dips**
- **Obtain youthful lustrous looks**
- **Firm up the neck and décolletage**
- **Diminish under eye bags**
- **Give your jaw line definition**
- **Have brighter eyes and better eyesight!**

Fitface is safe, affordable and feels good

Improved circulation from exercise brings more nutrients to the skin and also removes more internal toxins for a natural glow that is associated with youthful, healthy skin. Strong toned muscle tissue lifts and firms the whole face.

Why does most people's exercise routine stop at the neck, when they have seen proof "body" exercises work?

There are many reasons why facial exercises have not become popular. Personally, I believe it was because anyone caught doing them was branded a nut, a tree hugger, or new age. Now times and attitudes are changing, be it ever so slowly.

However, it is odd that "body exercise" really started to take off in the USA with Jack LaLanne. He pioneered so many fitness first's because he wanted to live life to the fullest. He was an avid fan of face exercises and incorporated them into his routines. He did not care that he was a man or looked stupid doing them on camera.

He had inner confidence and was proud of the way he looked and did not separate the body from the face. *Perhaps we have finally come full circle now as is often the case with history? Time will tell.*

It never ceases to amaze me (and responsible reporters of the global beauty trade) that although consumers are presented the facts about the serious side effects or risks a beauty product has that demand remains unchanged. Worse still that "positive news" outstrips "negative news" which is subsequently buried. They now do say, "Even bad news is good publicity" because it has a positive impact on the sales of products. This is especially true with anti-aging beauty products, notably with creams, whereby the consumer simply switches brands for a while.

For example:
Headlines: The Sun Newspaper December 24, 2011
Brit women beg private firms to remove boob implants
WOMEN are begging private cosmetic surgery firms to remove their toxic PIP implants — after French health authorities ordered surgeons to do the same. **The faulty implants were used in more than 40,000 British boob jobs.**

Nevertheless, just four months later!!!
Flat-chested mum and daughter get bust boosting boob jobs together
Seen on AOL UK 11 April 2101 Reported on Parent Dish
"We are both thrilled to bits with our new boobs - we just can't wait to go shopping for a whole new wardrobe of fancy bras and low cut tops"
http://www.parentdish.co.uk/2012/04/10/flat-chested-mum-and-daughter-get-bust-boosting-boob-jobs-together/?icid=maing-grid7%7Cuk%7Cdl6%7Csec1_lnk3%26pLid%3D103816

The manufacturers of beauty products know that women totally seem to disregard the truth when it comes to products offering eternal youth, and only want to be fed hopeful messages, even though they are false!

The consumer reasons

For every person, there is a reason for not doing facial exercise. the following are the most common ones I've encountered.

- **Fear of producing more static wrinkles**

That is just propaganda put out by the multimillion dollar cosmetic industry, but admittedly it's pretty persuasive. But, think about it logically. BOTOX® injections relax the muscle pull causing the wrinkle - and so does exercise - only naturally. Face exercise also strengthens the surrounding muscles; thereby you are working on more than one muscle at a time. Healthy, tight, toned muscles last a lifetime BOTOX® does not. Moreover, **BOTOX® promotes wrinkles because the surrounding unused muscles work to make an expression for which they were not naturally intended**. The truth is that facial exercise prevents wrinkles,

There is evidence that BOTOX® actually causes wrinkles. In a piece for the Journal of Cosmetic Dermatology in 2002, Dr David Becker, an assistant professor of dermatology at Weill Cornell Medical College in New York, observed that 'wrinkles caused by untreated muscles of facial expression paradoxically can become more prominent'.

The only thing I can say is for you to take a long hard look at the faces of those few people in the West like me who advocate facial exercises. Then ask yourself "If facial exercises cause wrinkles, then why don't they look awful? And furthermore, because they do facial exercises extensively, "Why don't their faces look horribly disfigured and lined with millions of wrinkles, far more so than the average person? In actual fact, "Why do these people look as good as, (and certainly more natural) than those persons who have had injections and knives at their faces for over the past 25 years?

I especially designed Fitface to be "hands free" because 25 years ago I too was afraid and thought that I might get more wrinkles. But, I had to wait a very long time almost 25 years) to find out that you don't and patience is not my strong point! I am glad they are "hands-free" as I still have an inherent objection to unnaturally pulling the skin on my face in every direction. However, I do think that the benefits of facials, massage or hands on exercise outweigh the possible negative impact.

There are still some people who just have blinkers on, which is fair enough. Once upon a time people once thought the earth was flat!

- **Time**

Until you really get used to doing facial exercises, they can be time consuming. However, once you have learned them by heart they then become "easy peasy, lemon squeezy!" Muscles learn and remember, unlike a visit to the salon.

Sometimes an urgent event has motivated a person to make a drastic change, to get a quick fix with an injection, or worse still a facelift. Facial exercises make a subtle lasting lifetime difference. Injections make a much bigger impression, not only in the short-term, but most especially over time, after the skin has become unbearably stretched from repeatedly sooner and sooner, more and more filler is needed to be injected under the skin to puff up ever thinning skin. Injections have become a way of life, a slippery downward cycle. The injections are required more frequently because the skin has been pumped up artificially and stretched - thinning the surface, which means the next result gives less improvement. A cycle of dependency begins, with ever decreasing results. The economic law of ever diminishing returns!

Fortunately, *(I do not think)* facelifts are undertaken lightly even by the very brave or stupid, but I have been asked what I would think of having one done in Thailand!! **PLEASE, PLEASE, PLEASE, DON'T** – unless of course, you live there. If you must have one done please be at home, wherever that may be, some place where you can conduct reliable research on the surgeon, etc. Then, if you do go ahead and if something does go wrong, you will then at least feel that you had tried to do your best and most importantly you will have your friends "at home" to support you.

There is **no going back from a facelift** and do bear in mind that you will probably need further surgeries in the future and perhaps other work such as a brow lift, cheek implants, etc. This is radical surgery, cutting healthy tissue with all of the associated risks. You have been warned.

- **Effort**

Learning anything takes time, dedication and effort. It is much easier to take your chance at the beauty salon, plus you can meet your friends, etc

Although I hate to be the bearer of bad tidings, like anything else you do in life; the result of the effort you put in generally pays dividends. Having the work/beauty stuff done for you is not quite the same, and the face knows! It would be like doing ordinary body exercises, but having someone else to lift up your back to do a sit up. You can't fool the body, or the face, it's just not quite the same!

There are no independent studies done, but I guess it's obvious, that exercise machines (be them electronic, electrical, photon, ultrasound or galvanic current) do not stimulate the face in the same way as face exercise. Furthermore, they are "involuntary muscle contractions;" (produced by artificially moving muscles) and are biologically different. The nerve ending signals travel a different route, to a different part of the brain, because the stimulation is not the same as voluntary face exercises. As a result the message to the brain is different/changed. *Perhaps that is the reason they do not work as well; is it because they got lost in translation?*

- **Belief in face creams**

There is an almost unfathomable belief that facial creams are somehow miraculous and are able to make unhealthy face skin glow. Some can help, but it is really daft to think that they can lift the muscles to take ten years off the face! They can only treat the surface. That is all they were designed to do. An over the counter cream cannot alter the skins structure, or **it would not be sold without a prescription.**

Regardless of previous information having been exposed about the false claims of various products produced by most major

French cosmetic company; the belief and hope of a brighter future, with NEW anti-aging "designer" creams remains prevalent.

I discussed this at length with a friend of mine who freely admitted that if the claim said it would make her look 10 years younger in three weeks, she would pay whatever. Perhaps, in real terms she'd pay £150 - £220 for a 4oz jar without giving a thought as to the cabinet at home full of previous purchased ineffectual and useless stuff! It is so sad but true!

However, I am pleased to write that there have been significant improvements in adding Vitamin C into skin care products. The old problem was that when vitamin C, was exposed to sunlight, it would degrade i.e. oxidise. Now, there are a new generation of vitamin C products with something added to stop this; hopefully they really may have overcome the problem? *Um, I'm not so sure, although I commend Dr. Bunting's warning that not all vitamin C creams are equal, that much is true.*

It would be nice to believe that scientists have also found that it actually kick starts the body into producing more collagen and elastin! Once again, when I read this and know that it is rubbish, (just a copy and paste job by an over stressed journalist, interested only in the primary objective of getting the column inches of copy produced to be able to collect a pay check). *Do I blame the journalist? Hell no; I would probably would do the same in their situation. I am only distressed that the readership buys into what is written.*

Generally, the real benefit of most creams is the extra circulation and hydration of the skin when the product is applied. Fitface is the natural beauty spa that achieves better toning and glowing results than any expensive cream with an ordinary light moisturiser. Fitface also has the additional hidden extra benefits of better eyesight and healthier hair, etc!

Would a daily vitamin pill do the job just as well? "No," according to dermatologist Dr. Sam Bunting who's studies show we can increase the amount of vitamin C in our skin simply through diet. "Sunlight and pollution deplete the skin's vitamin C supply so it makes sense to deliver it topically."

Great (if true) about the new vitamin C creams, but when you add something else unnatural to a product (probably a nasty chemical) all sorts of weird and wonderful things happen. The body naturally tries to combat the unnatural invader (which is how the skin responds to chemicals, believing the skin is under attack by a foreign invader) i.e. the product being put on our faces. *Hey, it's great if they work, and I would love to know more, so do write.*

The medical professions reason

Cosmetic surgeons

Make no mistake; Cosmetic Surgery is a business - with multimillion dollar turnovers for those businesses that get it right. Many have a network of locations; a sales force, call centres and all, are target driven. They offer you "free consultations" with a member of the sales team, who delivers the sales pitch, and introduces the various treatment packages. They even offer financial plans with options to pay over 5 years!

The doctors must come up with new products, and faster procedures, all designed to keep bringing the clients back for more. The doctors and staff make no secret or it, or apology for it. They freely admitted it was a business in **Bum, Boob and BOTOX®** a behind-the-scenes TV documentary about "Transform" the UK's biggest provider of Cosmetic Surgery.

I was shocked, amazed, flabbergasted at the flippant statements. Whilst I do understand I am anti their business and that surgery has moved on, I was completely stunned by the uptake of procedures by the potential patients from the call centres verbatim of chit chat about RADICAL SURGERY. Do these women not understand that these ladies at call canters are just: reading scripts? Do they not realize that these friendly ladies are not doctors, let alone cosmetic surgeons? Do they not know that these ladies are on a commission to sell as many procedures as they can? Do they not comprehend that the any injection into the skin or cutting of the skin could prove fatal? *I guess not? I can only imagine that the public feels so protected by the "State" (and able to sue if things go wrong or that things are not as purported to be what they believed to be true) that they are comfortable. The responsibility for their lives is in someone else's hands, I suppose I come from a different generation.*

I really have to give it to Transform, they were honest, and did not hold anything back; they even informed the audience that the clients get hooked when they see that the lines are coming back, saying that it was good news for them, it means repeat business. As they put it, "In today's market "is all about bringing back volume."

Times are changing elsewhere. At one time, the medical profession was publicly against facial exercises; but because cosmetic surgeons recommend some exercises after facial surgery, they are forced to concede and must agree that facial exercises build strong facial tissues and muscle.

Skin only facelifts that were once normal practice, are now considered archaic. Today, a SMAS facelift (rhytidectomy) involves a full muscular system lift all over the face where the work is done on the deepest (third) layer. This deep facelift surgical procedure is meant to reduce the appearance of sagging jowls, cheeks and neck skin. (Why not prevent them at the deepest level with exercise?).
http://en.wikipedia.org/wiki/Superficial_muscular_aponeurotic_system

The most honest and highly respected internationally renowned surgeon whom I spoke to told me that he "recommended facial exercise to his clients" and he would only perform surgery on his clients at an age when he felt facial exercise was not beneficial anymore. He obviously had an enormous client base. I have enormous respect for him.

The tide is turning and with all the work available I believe more cosmetic surgeons will start recommending them to their younger clients who are not, and never will be celebrities. However, it remains a 'conflict of interest' for most junior surgeons seeking a client base and the much older surgeons who are stuck in their ways.

On a personal note, I am not at all anti cosmetic surgeons. In my book Fitface 2, I describe how a team of surgeons saved my daughter's life and her face after a horrendous accident for which I am eternally grateful.

Medical doctors

Many younger doctors do see facial exercises as beneficial, but their older "bosses" in hospitals may not agree, therefore, they are reluctant to speak out. I cannot understand it - they promote body exercising for blood circulation– it makes no sense. Even if, the only benefit of facial exercising was a better supply of nutrients to the sense organs in the face and the hair, you would think they would agree with me, and the medical doctors that I talk with - perhaps in time?

My question to these doubting doctors would be, *"Why then are facial exercises recommended as a treatment for a patient suffering with Bell's palsy?* (Bell's palsy causes a drop to one side of the face). Surely, that advice would suggest that facial exercise can lift dropping sagging skin? Is that not what young women want to avoid (a droopy face) and older women want to cure?

Physiotherapy can be beneficial to some individuals with Bell's palsy as it helps to maintain muscle tone of the affected facial muscles and stimulate the facial nerve. It is important that muscle re-education exercises and soft tissue techniques be implemented prior to recovery in order to help prevent permanent contractures of the paralyzed facial muscles Muscle re-education exercises are also useful in restoring normal movement.
http://en.wikipedia.org/wiki/Bell's_palsy

Dermatologists

Simply put, it is a conflict of interest when it comes to beauty for those that gain most of their income from performing cosmetic procedures on patients and sales of cosmetic products. If a cream is prescribed as effective ask to see the clinical trial test results, this should be easy to locate if your dermatologist recommends it.

They are especially negative towards facial exercise practitioners, possibly because non "hands free" exercises could potentially stretch the skin, but mainly, I think, because we (myself and most others in my profession) educate the public about the ingredients in "special cosmetic creams." We explain that many cannot penetrate the outer skin layers and thus these creams are ineffectual. For example: collagen therefore it must be injected.

However, I was delighted to read that not all dermatologists are pro injections. For example:

Leading cosmetic dermatologist, Dr Nick Lowe, of the Cranley Clinic in London, says: 'If you inject the forehead with Botox, the muscles at the sides of the nose and on the lower bridge of the nose often act a bit more strongly, just because the adjacent muscles have been reduced in strength by the injections. That's why you get bunny lines. "Some people have them naturally, but increasingly, bunny lines are being seen as a dead giveaway that the person in question has submitted to the needle."
http://www.marieclaire.co.uk/news/health/454268/can-botox-give-you-wrinkles.html

The beauty industry reasons

If facial exercises were actually to really "catch on," potentially the beauty industry and related industries would lose billions. The market is enormous. Skin care is by far the most important category in the global beauty and personal-care industry, accounting for nearly a quarter of total sales in 2009. Anti-agers continue to be the star performer, showing consistently high increases in revenue over the last five years. Although growth slipped slightly to 7 percent in 2009 (down from 9% in 2008) it still far outperformed the overall global skin care category (3% growth) as well as the global beauty and personal care industry as a whole (4% growth).

Despite some trading down during the recession, premium skin care is set to see the biggest increase in value size of any premium segment, with US $2.6 billion set to be added over 2009 to 2014, equating to 40 percent of absolute growth in the entire premium beauty industry. This performance will be driven by strong demand for premium anti-agers in Asia, especially China.

Even in Western markets like the United States, sales of high-end anti-agers have remained comparatively buoyant as consumers have evidently attached **greater importance to fighting the aging process than other areas of beauty and personal care, and the perception of a link between price and efficacy remains strong for many consumers despite evidence to the contrary.**
Future growth in the skin-care category will continue to be driven by anti-agers.
http://www.insidecosmeceuticals.com/articles/2011/02/global-cosmeceuticals-market.aspx

Spas

These are wonderful places for making you feel magnificent and stress free, all good for the circulation of the skin, relaxing the mind, rejuvenating the body and lifting the spirits. However, there is once again a conflict of interest, in as much as they provide a service and sell all sorts of face creams. They want and need you to come back for another treatment, preferably a weekly facial at the minimum price, or better still a monthly maintenance treatment. And when at home; they prefer you to use their personally branded products (that they have either have had privately labelled for their salon) or those for which they are licensed agents to sell (usually an expensive brand name only available at special beauty salons). They do not want you staying at home with a cheap supermarket moisturiser and face exercise book!

Treatments are big business with all sorts of new ones coming in and going out of fashion. Even facials are not cheap, for example a "geisha treatment" (nightingale's poo facial) can be $200 in New York. The procedures now offered at many spas have expanded into using an array of gadgets and machines which offer other opportunities for profit. The procedures offered have become more invasive such as chemical peels and some spas (now called Medical spas) have even crossed the line into offering a selection of invasive procedures such as fillers by injections.

It's worrying to think that a girl can go on a weekend course and then inject something into someone's face that may have serious side effects. One college proudly advertises its courses by saying that they provide the most training in the industry: **"hands-on experience (over 5 hours of live patient injections) on their one day course.** Ah, that perhaps explains why the accidental deaths from injections have occurred at non medical facilities as there had not been time to rush the victim to hospital. Hopefully the LAW may be changing, the subject is being debated.
http://www.consultingroom.com/blog/Display.asp?Blog_ID=163

In the States, I was in talks with a group about setting up classes in a Woman's Health Centre before I had to fly home to take care of my mother. Now that she is better I should probably rethink that idea, but maybe instead, here in the UK.

Cosmeceuticals & pharmaceutical companies

Maintaining or recovering a youthful appearance is a multibillion dollar industry driven by the desire for healthy great looking-skin – regardless of age. Facial exercises are of no commercial value to them and as a result billions would be lost in revenue.

Cosmeceutical companies

Cosmeceuticals refers to the combination of cosmetics and pharmaceuticals. Cosmeceuticals are cosmetic products with biologically active ingredients purporting to have medical or drug-like benefits.

Dermatological research suggests that the bioactive ingredients used in cosmeceuticals have benefits beyond the traditional moisturiser However, despite reports of benefits from some cosmeceutical products, there are no requirements to prove that these products live up to their claims. The "cosmeceutical" label applies only to products applied topically, such as creams, lotions, and ointments.

The term "cosmeceutical" is often used in cosmetic advertising, and may be misleading to the consumer. If the consumer interprets a cosmeceutical to be similar to a pharmaceutical product, he or she may conclude that cosmeceuticals are required to undergo the same testing for efficacy and quality control as required for medication. This may allow the retailer to charge the consumer more for a product which may actually be less effective and/or of poorer quality than perceived. The reputation of the product may be falsely enhanced if the consumer incorrectly believes that a "cosmeceutical" is held to the same FDA standards as a drug.
http://en.wikipedia.org/wiki/Cosmeceutical

Pharmaceutical companies

It's all about money. Facial exercises are in direct competition with injectable fillers and/or a neurotoxin such as BOTOX® (Botulinum toxin is the most powerful yet discovered).
http://en.wikipedia.org/wiki/Neurotoxin

January 18, 2012—Toronto—According to Millennium Research Group (MRG), the global authority on medical technology market intelligence, the North American facial injectables market will see strong growth through 2016, despite significant downward pressure on selling prices caused by the entry of new, lower-priced products into the market. Growth will average 11 percent per year, and the market will grow from $844 million in 2011 to more than $1.4 billion in 2016.

The media
(Journalists, TV/radio/magazines + the supporting industries and contributors)

Beauty products are reported by the media on TV, radio, in print, and on-line. The very existence and survival of the media companies depend almost entirely on revenues generated by advertising. Therefore, they either produce glowing propaganda filled with beauty articles/editorials and advertisements to suit the desires of their paying clients or allow inclusion of them. It pays the bills! Most mass consumer media publications are not in the business of putting the interests of their reader's first or educating the public to empower them with knowledge detrimental to their income.

Journalists do care *(I hope)* about what they write/report, but there are simply only so many hours in a day. These journalists are experts in every field, only a few are investigative reporters, producing copy or a TV show to uncover some hidden untruth not yet disclosed. Even then - we may only watch in awe, momentarily riveted in disgust, but seldom do such documentaries really produce change. Such is my quest with Fitface.

Journalists have a contract to fill and a job to do; they cannot possibly be expected to know about everything even in their field, for example; fashion and makeup. Their job is to report trends, what's in and what's out, what sells and what doesn't, what's hot and what is not. They are not ultimately responsible for misinformation; they report what they hear and perhaps neither are the editors who get the information from the journalists. Even if there were someone to blame we all know that they too have bosses, shareholders or zillionaire's objectives to fulfil. *I am not being cynical, just real. Why would the media bite the hand that feeds it?*

The "others"

There are millions of people employed worldwide in the billion dollar beauty industry

Chapter 3

Key biological facts
Wrinkles - Formation and the different types
Muscles – How they move and grow
Skin, collagen and elastin

If you desire a healthy, great looking radiant skin regardless of your age, all you really need to know: is that
exercise is good for you
too good for you to stop at the neck
exercise your face too!

Skin grows from the inside out

Skip this chapter if you like; but if nothing else it's fun and interesting to see how the muscles move under your skin.

Muscles of Facial Expression
Anatomy Tutorial
http://www.youtube.com/watch?v=Xmz3oLrnzBw

Artnatomy
Anatomical basis of facial expression learning tool
http://www.artnatomia.net/uk/index.html

The basics

Think of the face as a "facemask" extending down the neck. This facemask is a web of muscular fibres, a skin covering of about 1.3mm thick (thinnest on the eyelids).

The facial muscles are a group of striated muscles innervated by the facial nerve that, among other things, control facial expression. These muscles are also called mimetic muscles.

The top layer of this mask is dead skin and to function as protection from the elements. The middle layer of the mask is the substance (collagen and elastin proteins) - the layer where new skin cells are manufactured. The final and last layer is fat to cushion and protect.

The facemask web is attached to the skull at the forehead and held down at the back of the neck by another huge muscular skin covering, shaped like a Roman helmet. This covering is attached at different points on the skull bone by muscles. Therefore, basically the whole head is covered in muscular fibre; therefore it makes perfect sense to exercise it.

In the body most of the skeletal muscles are internal under the skin and fat, attached bone on bone.

Anatomically

The muscles of facial expression are very superficial (being attached to or influencing the skin) and are all supplied with information by the facial nerve. In addition to those of the scalp and auricle (ear), muscles are arranged around the openings of the eyes, nose, and mouth.

SMAS is an acronym for Superficial Muscular Aponeurotic System. It refers to an area of musculature of the face. The SMAS is a connected system of muscles and collagen-rich connective tissue responsible for smiling, frowning and other facial expressions.

This muscular system is manipulated during facial cosmetic surgery, especially rhytidectomy (facelift). The SMAS extends

from the Platysma (neck) to the Galea Aponeurotica (forehead) and is continuous with Temporoparietal Fascia (temples and above ear) and Galea. It connects to the dermis via vertical septa).
en.wikipedia.org/wiki/Superficial_muscular_aponeurotic_system

Galea Aponeurotica
The "galea aponeurotica" is a long-winded word for the muscle which covers the upper part of the cranium (skull). Its' attachment to the frontal and occipital bellies (muscles on the brow at the front and on the upper back of the head) allows it to move the scalp freely over the underlying skull bone.
http://www.innerbody.com/image_musfov/musc16-new.html

An overview of wrinkle formation and how to erase them

Facial muscles are contracted to form an expression.

The muscles are attached to the underside of the skin and when contracted - pull the skin down causing a groove. A crease is made, a slight pull inwards, a wrinkle.

With constant contractions of a specific facial muscle (to form a particular facial expression), the muscle used the most (exercised) becomes strong, stronger the strongest muscle. That muscle, overtime, becomes the most powerful, dominant muscle; pulling on the skin to form the required facial expression. For example: a frown.

All the other facial muscles learn to cooperate with each other and work in sync to help form the desired facial expression (such as when you learned to walk – it's no good one foot going sideways when the leg wants to go forward!).

In the face, over time and with constant repetitive movements to form a specific facial expression (such as a frown) the dominate muscle prevails. The surrounding muscles weaken in compliance with the desired expression (through lack of use). Unused they relax, weaken and eventually give up working.

The dominant muscle gains ever more strength over many years and becomes ever stronger and holds tight, tighter and it does not relax its grip or dominance; eventually over time a deep, deeper grove/wrinkle is formed. Therefore, even at rest the muscles cleverly produce the expression most asked for, - be it a frown!

The rest of the facial tissues follow suit. The facia within the SMAS (consists of a dense mesh of **collagen**, elastic, and muscle fibres) becomes depressed by the constant pulling action and are compressed. Over time this covering literally becomes "stuck in the groove."

There are two methods to loosen, relax and unstick a static wrinkle:

Naturally with exercise

To solve three problems at once, the muscles and the fascia (collagen/elastin) issues
- the surrounding muscles can be strengthened - to pull up and out the wrinkle
- to produce an increase in collagen (within the fascia) - to replace the lost squashed out collagen to plump the wrinkle out
- Lasts a lifetime (remember muscles learn)

Unnaturally with injections

To solve one problem at a time
- Inject a toxic poison into the muscle which will block messages from the brain to tell the muscle not to work. The muscle is in effect paralysed. Repeat every 3 - 6 months.
However neurotoxins MIGRATE and spread. Without working any muscles in that area they all become weak. Guess what happens to skin unsupported by muscle – that's right it sags. Now it's filler time!
- Inject a filler or fillers, preferably a natural source of collagen, (better still if it is from the patient and not a cow) under the skin to replace and puff up the lost collagen. By repeating the process and adding a little more filler each time as the skin stretches beyond the original wrinkle.

Radically with surgery

Pull back the muscular skin covering that covers the face this will also pull up the muscles, cut away excess healthy skin tissue and pull taut. Attach the SMAS to the helmet like muscular covering of the skull and fasten with stitches.

The problem is that when one introduces anything artificial into the face (like filler) or body there are unnatural consequences and a price to pay. Overtime the wrinkles will come back, quicker than the lifetime it took to get them there before because the faces' intricate balance has been disrupted and skin has thinned, become weakened thus damaged.

Overtime with even more procedures the natural appearance of the subject becomes distorted, plastic, unreal, and slightly odd. Unfortunately the patient often becomes physiologically addicted to chasing the dream with ever diminishing results. Sadly the patients become deformed achieving the exact opposite of their most wanted desire. (More later in Chapter 4).

Before discussing the numerous benefits of facial exercise or the alternatives further, let me give you a brief overview of what matters to you about the anatomy of the face. However, I would be the first to admit that it is very complex and when it comes to muscles and how they work; it gets worse, and yes even more confusing. Throughout this section I have tried to condense the vast amount of sometimes conflicting information and only leave in the salient points, and please feel free to skip bits or conversely research more. Perhaps you can find a medical paper that I am not aware of and if so please do write to me for inclusion in Fitface 4 for which I would be delighted to credit you for.

There are three forms of wrinkles

- Static wrinkles – wrinkles visible at rest
- Dynamic – wrinkles are only visible when the face is animated
- Wrinkle folds

Static wrinkles

Static wrinkles are the wrinkles and folds that are present at rest or when we are not forming facial expressions. They develop as we get older because natural substances such as collagen, elastin and hyaluronic acid that provide the skin with structure and volume decrease with age. The loss of skin structure and volume means that the skin is less able to spring back to its initial position after facial expression, and as a result static wrinkles and folds form.

Examples of static wrinkles:
- The crêpe like skin around the eyes that usually begins in the mid 30s and continues to progress with age
- That crosshatched appearance of the skin around the cheek areas that starts to show up in the late 30s and gets progressively more pronounced with age

Dynamic wrinkles

Occur when we use our muscles to form facial expressions. During facial expressions such as smiling and frowning our muscles contract and cause our skin to wrinkle. For example, when we smile our eye wrinkles become prominent and when we frown the vertical lines between our eyebrows become noticeable. When we are young our skin springs back to its original position when we finish making the facial expression (at rest) but as we get older, very gradually the dynamic wrinkles remain on the skin to form static wrinkles.

Examples of dynamic wrinkles
- Frowning or furrowing the brow contracts certain muscles that create those deep **static** wrinkle lines between the eyebrows.
- Raising of the eyebrows contracts muscles that, over time, etch those horizontal wrinkle lines across the forehead.
- Smiling and squinting bunch the skin on the cheeks and near the outer corners of the eyes, making the wrinkled lines we commonly refer to as crow's feet.

Wrinkle folds

The third types of wrinkles are referred to as wrinkle folds. In most cases, wrinkle folds are caused by the loss of subcutaneous facial fat and sagging of the underlying facial structures. This is truly the most common type of wrinkles from the natural progression of age.
http://tracey-drake.suite101.com/3-wrinkle-types-associated-with-body-aging-a154817

How the body works

Research into tissue growth and repair represents a wide-ranging and exciting research direction especially with new further developments in genetics. There are a large number of scientists in different parts of the world working to better understand the role of a range of tissues and organ systems. How the cells work within the various muscles tissues and how the largest organ in the body, the skin works remains for the most part a mystery.

A mini biology lesson

How muscles grow

Muscle growth is an extremely complex molecular biological cell process involving the interplay of numerous cellular organelles and growth factors, occurring as a result of exercise. Muscle growth is a vastly researched topic yet still considered a fertile area of research.

There are two ways in which muscles grow

- **Hypertrophy**
- **Hyperplasia**

Muscle **hypertrophy** is an increase in the **size** of muscle cells. Muscle **hyperplasia** is the formation of **new** muscle cells.

ADAPTIVE CELL CHANGES

Normal Cells

Nucleus

Hypertrophy

Basement Memebrane

Hyperplasia

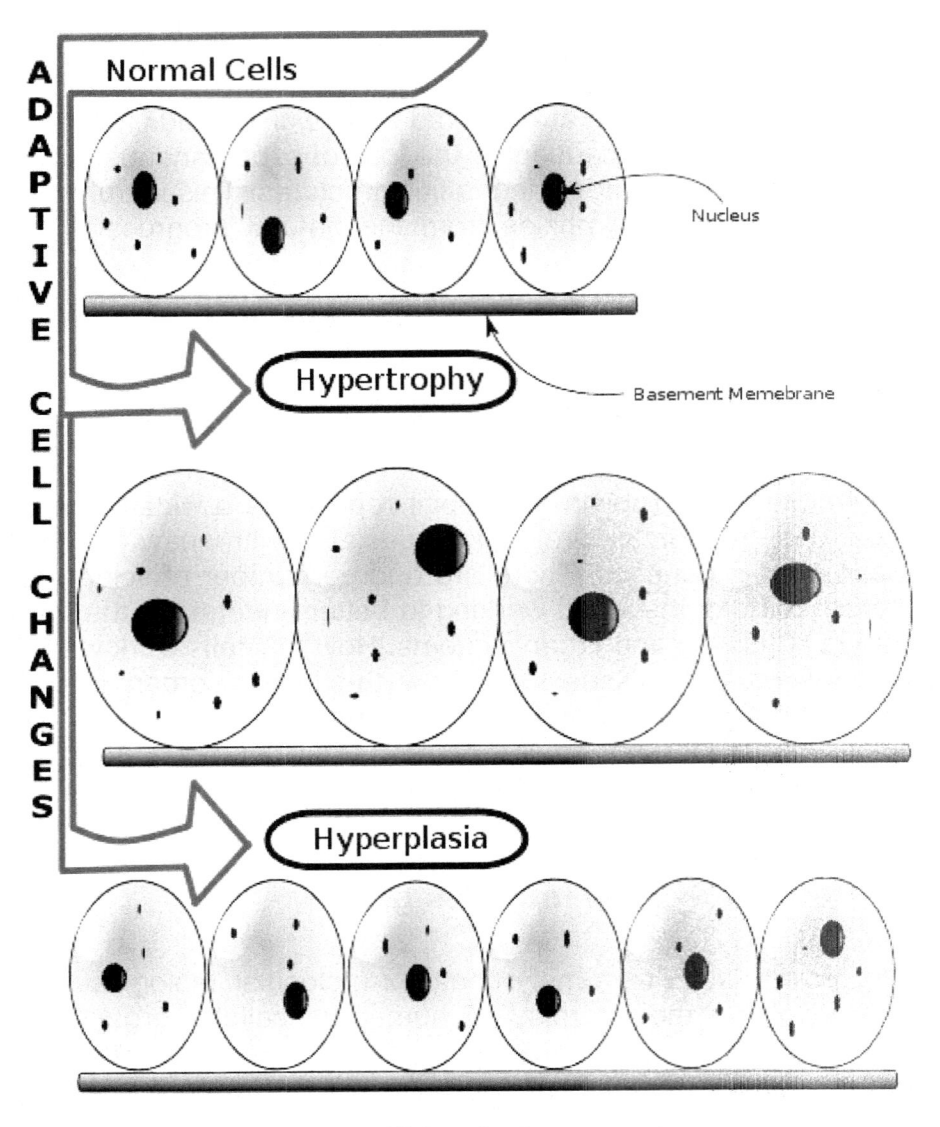

http://en.wikipedia.org/wiki/Muscle_hypertrophy
http://en.wikipedia.org/wiki/Hyperplasia
http://en.wikipedia.org/wiki/Cell_proliferation

Muscle Hyperplasia (or "hypergenesis") means increase in number of cells

Animal tests have shown that stretching a muscle can trigger hyperplasia, **though this phenomenon has yet to be confirmed in humans. Hyperplasia may** also be induced through specific power output training for athletic performance, thus increasing the number of muscle fibres instead of increasing the size of a single fibre. An example of normal Hyperplasia is the increase in breast size. in pregnancy.

Hyperplasia may also be **induced artificially by injecting hormones** such as IGF-1 and human growth hormone. Perhaps the most interesting and potent effect IGF has on the human body is its ability to cause hyperplasia, which is an actual splitting of cells. The term **steroid** describes both hormones produced by the body and artificially produced medications that duplicate the action for the naturally occurring steroids.

As adults we cannot produce new muscles fibres readily and when they are gone – they're gone for good. The growth of new muscle cells and their development into muscle fibres, if such a phenomenon exists we would be discussing myofibril hyperplasia. Whilst we cannot easily produce new muscles cells, we can however change the size of the cells we've got.

Muscle hypertrophy is an increase in the size of muscle cells.

Resistance training (in face pull against attachment to the skin) leads to trauma or injury of the cellular proteins in muscle. This prompts cell-signalling messages to activate satellite cells to begin a cascade of events leading to muscle growth and repair.

> Therefore, when you train your muscles and they get bigger, **(you are not actually growing new muscles cells -hyperplasia).**

Instead each individual muscle cell grows in size (hypertrophy) to help your body cope with increases in muscle loading as an adaptive response that serves to increase the ability to generate force or resist fatigue in anaerobic conditions.

Muscle hypertrophy is caused by an increase in the number and size of myofibrils per muscle cell, increased total protein (especially myosin), and increased amounts of connective tissue (tendons and ligaments).

Inside your muscle cells, there is **sarcoplasm** (a fluid) and myofibrils (one of the slender threads of a muscle fibre).

- The best way to make your muscles grow bigger is to increase the sarcoplasm by **fatigue/repetitions** in your muscles.
- The best way to make your muscles grow stronger is to increase the density of myofibrils with **weights**.

How muscle hypertrophy works
- Exercise leads to trauma or injury of the cellular proteins in muscle
- This prompts cell-signalling messages to activate satellite cells to begin a cascade of events leading to muscle repair and growth

Aging also mediates cellular changes in muscle decreasing the actual muscle mass. This loss of muscle mass is referred to as **sarcopenia**. Happily, the detrimental effects of aging on muscle have been shown to be restrained or even reversed with regular resistance exercise.

www.unm.edu/~lkravitz/Article%20folder/musclesgrowLK.html

How muscles move

Muscle fibre generates tension through the action of actin and myosin cross-bridge cycling. While under tension, the muscle may lengthen, shorten, or remain the same. Although the term contraction implies shortening, when referring to the muscular system, it means muscle fibres generating tension with the help of motor neurons (the terms twitch tension, twitch force, and fibre contraction are also used).

Fitface face exercises are voluntary muscle movements

Voluntary muscle contraction is controlled by the central nervous system. The brain sends signals, in the form of action potentials, through the nervous system to the motor neuron that innervates several muscle fibres. In the case of some reflexes, the signal to contract can originate in the spinal cord through a feedback loop with the grey matter.

Involuntary muscles such as the heart or smooth muscles in the gut and vascular system contract as a result of **non-conscious**

brain activity or stimuli proceeding in the body to the muscle itself.
http://en.wikipedia.org/wiki/Muscle_contraction
http://www.brianmac.co.uk/mustrain.htm

Classification of voluntary muscular contractions

Skeletal muscle contractions can be broadly separated into twitch and "**tetanic" contractions**.

In a twitch contraction, a short burst of stimulation causes the muscle to contract, but the duration is so short that the muscle begins relaxing before reaching peak force.

This occurs when a muscle's motor unit is stimulated at a sufficiently high frequency of multiple impulses. Each stimulus causes a twitch.

- If stimuli are delivered slow enough, the tension in the muscle will relax between successive twitches
- If stimuli are delivered at high frequency, then the twitches will add up, resulting in **tetanic contraction**. When tetanised, the contracting tension in the muscle remains constant in a steady state. This is the maximal contraction.

Voluntary muscular contractions can be further classified according to either length changes or force levels. In spite of the fact that the muscle actually shortens only in concentric contractions, all are typically referred to as "contractions."

- In concentric contraction
  The force generated is sufficient to overcome the resistance and the muscle shortens as it contracts.
  This is what most people think of as a muscle contraction.

- In eccentric contraction
  The force generated is insufficient to overcome the external load on the muscle and the muscle fibres lengthen as they contract.
  An eccentric contraction is used as a means of **decelerating** a body part or object, or lowering a load gently rather than letting it drop.

- In isometric contraction
  The muscle remains the same length.
  An example would be holding an object up without moving it; the muscular force precisely matches the load, and no movement results.

- In isotonic contraction
  The tension in the muscle remains constant despite a change in muscle length. This can occur only when a muscle's maximal force of contraction exceeds the total load on the muscle.

- In isovelocity contraction (sometimes called "isokinetic")
  The muscle contraction velocity remains constant, while force is allowed to vary.

  True isovelocity contractions are rare in the body, and are primarily an analysis method used in experiments on isolated muscles that have been dissected out of the organism. In reality; muscles rarely perform under any sort of constant force, velocity, or speed.
  wikipedia.org/wiki/Muscle_contraction#Eccentric_contraction

For Fitface I wanted readers to understand how the face, skin, and muscles interplay and what happens when, it is a very complex physiological process and not readily understood even by the experts. So once again if you want to skip this part do. Just remember, face exercises are good for you.

Contractions
- Isotonic (meaning same tension)
- Isometric (meaning same distance or not moving)

Isotonic Contractions

Isotonic contractions are those which cause the muscle to **change length** as it contracts and causes movement of a body part.

A muscular contraction in which the muscle remains to be in a **relatively constant tension** - while its length changes.

Isotonic movement, contractions

In almost every situation, everyday, we perform isotonic movements. In these types of movements we pick up a fixed weight, an empty pan, basically - anything that has weight. The weight of the pan is fixed but we decide how fast to lift it. We can lift it slowly, fast, or anywhere in between. The key to this type of movement is we decide how fast it goes but the weight (resistance) remains constant.
http://www.isokinetics.net/isokinetics/definitions/what-is-isokinetic.html

There are two types of isotonic contractions:

- **Concentric**
- **Eccentric**

Concentric contractions

Are those contractions which cause the muscle **to shorten** as it contracts. (The external force on the muscle is less than the force the muscle is generating – a shortening contraction).

Concentric contractions are the most common type of muscle contraction and occur frequently in daily and sporting activities.

Example: Bending the elbow from straight to fully flexed, causing a concentric contraction of the Biceps Brachii muscle.

Eccentric contractions

Are the opposite of concentric contractions and occur when the muscle **lengthens** as it contracts.

During an eccentric contraction, the muscle **elongates** while under tension due to an opposing force being greater than the force generated by the muscle.

Rather than working to pull a joint in the direction of the muscle contraction, the muscle acts to decelerate at the end of a movement or otherwise control the repositioning of a load. Eccentric contractions normally occur as a braking force in opposition to a concentric contraction to protect joints from damage. During virtually any routine movement, eccentric contractions assist in keeping motions smooth, but can also slow rapid movements such as a punch or throw.

Example: Kicking a football, the quadriceps muscle contracts concentrically to straighten the knee and the hamstrings contract eccentrically to decelerate the motion
www.teachpe.com/anatomy/types_of_muscle_contractions.php

Advantage
- Strengthens a muscle throughout the range of movement

Disadvantages
- Can make muscles sore, because of stress while they shorten
- The muscle gains most strength at the weakest point of the action, rather than evenly throughout

Isometric Contractions

An **isometric contraction** of a muscle generates force without changing length.

The joint angle **and the muscle length do not change** during contraction (compared to concentric/eccentric contractions called dynamic isotonic movements).

In isometric contractions, the muscle contracts but does not shorten, giving no movement.

Examples: "The Plank" in Pilates or the gripping of a tennis racket handle.

Advantages
- Isometric exercises develop static strength - the strength you need to push or pull a heavy object or hold it up
- They are quick to do and don't hurt
- They do not need expensive equipment
- You can do them anywhere

Disadvantages
- The muscle gains strength only at the angle you use in the exercise
- During an exercise, the blood flow to the muscle stops, blood pressure rises, and less blood flows back to the heart
- Isometric training is not sufficient on its own. You need to combine it with isotonic training

http://www.brianmac.co.uk/mustrain.htm
/en.wikipedia.org/wiki/Muscle_contraction#Concentric_contraction

NASA has researched the use of isometrics in preventing muscle atrophy experienced by astronauts as a result of living in a zero gravity environment. Isometrics, muscle lengthening and muscle shortening exercises were studied and compared.

The outcome showed that while all three exercise types of exercises did indeed promote muscle growth, isometrics failed to prevent a decrease in the amount of contractile proteins found in the muscle tissue. The result was muscle degradation at a molecular level. As contractile proteins are what cause muscles to contract and give them their physical strength; NASA has concluded that isometrics may not be the best way for astronauts to maintain muscle tissue.

http://en.wikipedia.org/wiki/Isometric_exercise

My best facial exercise theory

A high level of tension generates the signals for muscle strengthening.
- high levels of tension **can occur in both:**
    - isotonic eccentric contractions, and
    - isometric exercise - however - contractile proteins are not generated.

http://en.wikipedia.org/wiki/Isotonic_(exercise_physiology)

In conclusion:

I believe that the best facial movement exercise routine would be a combination of Isometric and Isotonic exercises (almost impossible in the face) concentrating on eccentric contractions to lengthen muscles.

Back to the gym! Do you remember how the fitness instructor would say, "Release slowly" and that the "letting go" (eccentric contractions) was as important as the lift? Well it seems that it is true.

A perfect exercise for the face would therefore be:

Warm up and wiggle your face and neck, (all your facial muscles) to get all the blood, nutrients and oxygen flowing.
Note: That it will take longer to stretch the facial muscles, either the tenser or the more familiar you are with facial exercise.
When you exercise a particular muscle, **concentrate.**
- Voluntarily move/contract a specific facial muscle and then hold the movement, tighten, tighter and then, release the muscle slowly a little, a little more, then let go.

Important information pertaining to facial muscles

Most muscles in the face:
- Are attached at one end to the underside of your skin
- Blend and inter-cross with another muscle
  Therefore, move one muscle and you move several muscles

It's a bit like learning to breath correctly, the sucking in is easy but the long exhale seems more difficult.

Muscles learn

Most of our actions, including the function of staying alive are controlled automatically by the sub conscious mind. That way the conscious mind is freed up of repetitive tasks. For the most part our body is "in sync" - working on auto pilot. This highly sophisticated mechanism explains how, for example, a professional tennis player is able to position themselves ready for the next 'shot' before their opponent has hit a return. In real time, a normal consciously functioning brain would not be able to compute the moves within the necessary nanoseconds but the unconscious automatic brain can. The muscles have learnt what they need to do when; they all work in sync after years of practice. Practice makes perfect.BBC 2 - Horizon.

Out of Control Episode 10 first aired March 13 2012
http://www.bbc.co.uk/programmes/b01dlglq

The skin

Diagram labels: hair shaft, sweat pore, dermal papilla, sensory nerve ending for touch, stratum corneum, pigment layer, stratum germinativum, stratum spinosum, stratum basale, arrector pili muscle, sebaceous gland, hair follicle, papilla of hair, nerve fiber, blood and lymph vessels, sweat gland, pacinian corpuscle, EPIDERMIS, DERMIS, SUBCUTIS (hypodermis), vein, artery

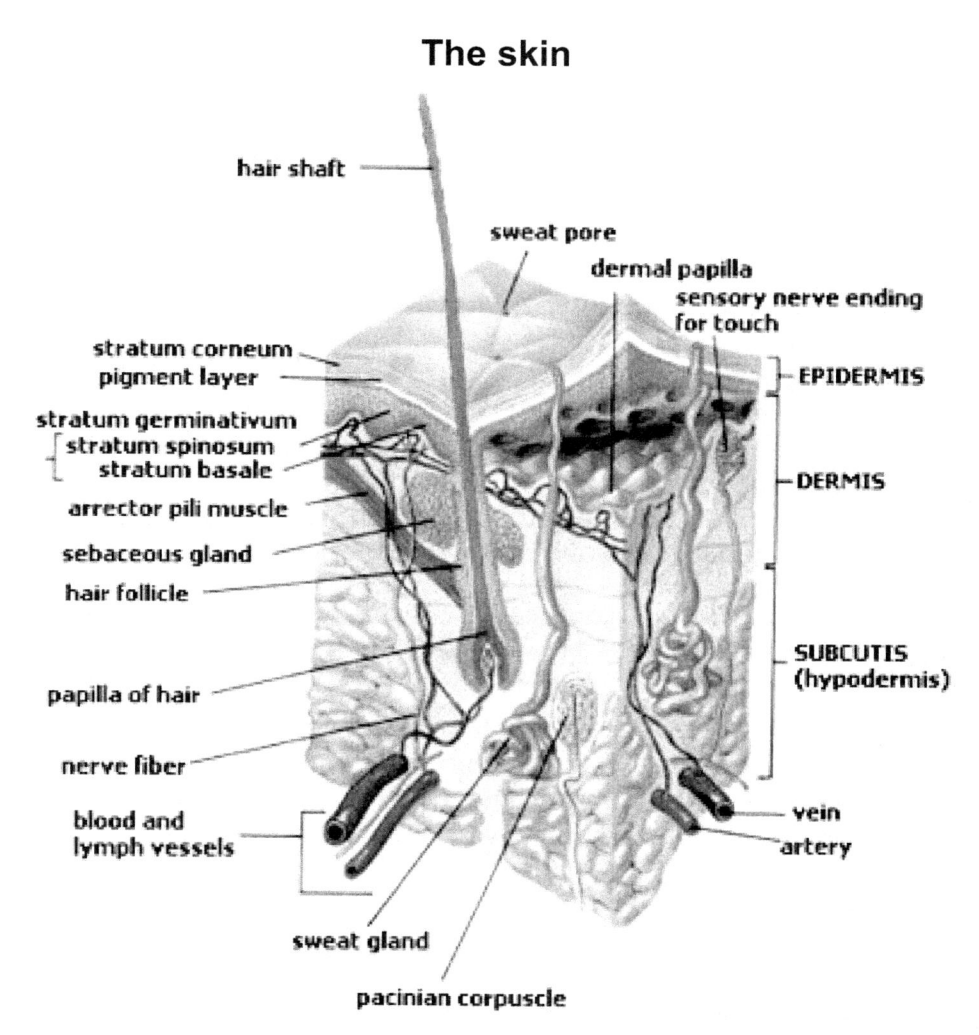

http://en.wikipedia.org/wiki/File:Skin.jpg

The skin is the surface covering of the body that protects it and receives external sensory stimuli, consisting of an epidermis over a thicker dermis. The epidermis contains cells involved in immune defences, sensory receptors, pigment cells, and keratin-producing cells. The last harden and migrate to the surface to form a dead, relatively dry outer layer of horny tissue that are constantly sloughs away, less often with advancing age.
http://www.answers.com/topic/skin#ixzz1rqDQr2Ya

The human skin is composed of three different layers.
1. **Epidermis**
2. **The Dermis**
3. **Subcuitis** (aka hypodermis, hypoderm, subcutaneous tissue, or superficial fascia)

Collectively known as the integumentary system; the skin is considered an organ, the largest of the body. Without it, living would be impossible. It holds moisture in the body, regulates temperature, acts as a protective layer against the outside world and contains many sensory nerves to warn you of dangerous conditions you may encounter.

Skin thickness

The thickness of the skin is a widely used parameter to evaluate the influence of various factors on skin aging. Skin thickness is significantly higher on the upper lip and lower lips, chin and infaobrital (beneath or below the eye socket) regions than on the forehead and cheeks.

Facial Skin

Facial skin has the same basic components as body skin with some minor differences. Facial skin has a thinner fat layer than the skin of the body. It can range from a fraction of an inch in the facial area to two or more inches in the abdominal area.

Women have smooth facial skin as opposed to more rugged in men. However, men have hair follicles where women have next to none. Wrinkles are more prominent on the face and neck than the rest of the body due to the thinner fat layer.
http://www.livestrong.com/article/174578-the-structure-of-human-skin-on-the-face-and-body/

Epidermis

The epidermis is the outer layer of skin. The thickness of the epidermis varies in different types of skin. It is the thinnest on the eyelids at .05 mm and the thickest on the palms and soles at 1.5 mm.

The epidermis contains 5 layers. From bottom to top the layers are named:

Stratum

- Comeum
- Lucidum (only present in thick skin – soles of feet)
- Granulosum
- Spinosum
- Basale

Section of epidermis

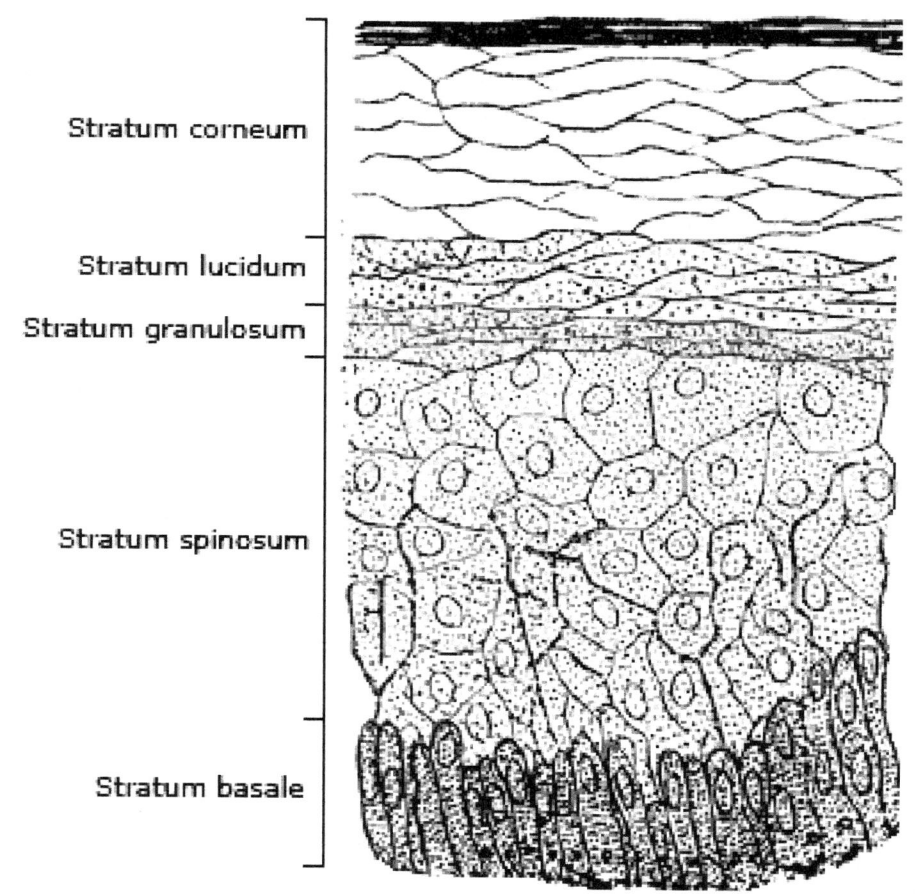

Stratum corneum
Stratum lucidum
Stratum granulosum
Stratum spinosum
Stratum basale

http://en.wikipedia.org/wiki/Stratum_spinosum

The epidermis contains no blood vessels and is entirely dependent on the underlying dermis for nutrient delivery and waste disposal via diffusion through the dermoepidermal junction.

Skin regeneration

Skin cells are constantly being born all the time in the middle skin layer, the dermis and are rising into the epidermal layers of the skin. They travel upwards and until they reach the surface where they are sloughed off.

Their journey upwards from birth to death takes anywhere from 14 – 35 days to complete. Young skin regenerates its surface area every two to three weeks on the epidermal layer. Older skin takes longer and longer to "slough off" dead cells. This shedding is natural. Exfoliation is an unnatural way of achieving this in older skin.

A good site to watch this in action is L'Oreal
http://www.skin-science.com/_int/_en/topic/topic_sousrub.aspx?tc=SKIN_SCIENCE_ROOT%5EAN_ORGAN_REVEALED%5ETHE_EPIDERMIS&cur=THE_EPIDERMIS

In biological terms, the epidermis is a stratified, squamous epithelium that consists primarily of keratinocytes in progressive stages of differentiation from deeper to more superficial layers.

- **The Stratum Corneum**
  Is the outermost layer of the skin. This layer contains almost entirely dead cells.

- **Stratum Granulosum** (or **granular layer**)
  The stratum granulosum creates a waterproof barrier between the outer layers of dead cells and the inner, live cells.

  This is the portion of the skin that is responsible for the skin's ability to stretch. The stratum granulosum is also known as the granular layer of the skin. This layer contains a protein that is responsible for the breakdown of skin cells.

- **Stratum Spinosum**
  This layer is also referred to as the "spinous" or "prickle-cell" layer because of the presence of cells with spiny arms diverging outward and interconnecting with other prickle cells. Generally, it is composed mainly of basal cells that are produced in the stratum basale and pushed upward to form prickle cells. These cells manufacture bipolar lipids that are organized into layers. The layers provide a structure that prevents evaporation of water and allows the skin to retain moisture.

- **Stratum Basale**
  The bottom layer has cells that are shaped like columns. In this layer the cells divide and push already formed cells into higher layers. As the cells move into the higher layers, they flatten and eventually die.

Dermis

The dermis layer contains blood vessels, nerve endings, deep sensory receptors, hair follicles, sweat glands, sebaceous glands and the erector pilli muscle that makes the hair stand on end. It is composed of **collagen** a type of connective tissue.

According to Holistic Online, the health of the collagen determines the health of the skin. Collagen holds moisture and prevents wrinkles. As you age, collagen and elastin deteriorates causing poor skin, sags and wrinkles.
http://www.livestrong.com/article/174578-the-structure-of-human-skin-on-the-face-and-body/#ixzz1rB9UNsYI

The primary function of the dermis is to sustain and support the epidermis. The dermis is a more complex structure and is composed of 2 layers - the more superficial papillary dermis and the deeper reticular dermis.
- **Papillary dermis** is thinner, consisting of loose connective tissue containing capillaries, elastic fibres, reticular fibres, and some **collagen**.
- **Reticular dermis** consists of a thicker layer of dense connective tissue containing larger blood vessels, closely

interlaced elastic fibres, and coarse bundles of collagen fibres arranged in layers parallel to the surface.

The **reticular** layer also contains fibroblasts, mast cells, nerve endings, lymphatics, and epidermal appendages. Surrounding the components of the dermis is the gel-like ground substance, composed of mucopolysaccharides (primarily hyaluronic acid), chondroitin sulfates, and glycoproteins. The deep surface of the dermis is highly irregular and borders the subcutaneous layer, the panniculus adiposus, which additionally cushions the skin.
http://emedicine.medscape.com/article/1294744-overview#aw2aab6b4

The **reticular** dermis is the lower layer of the dermis, found under the papillary dermis, composed of dense irregular connective tissue featuring densely packed collagen fibres (more later in this chapter). It is the primary location of dermal elastic fibres.
http://en.wikipedia.org/wiki/Reticular_dermis

The Subcutis (Subcutaneous fatty tissue)

The hypodermis, also called the hypoderm, subcutaneous tissue, or superficial fasciais the lowermost layer of the integumentary system invertebrates. It consists of spongy connective tissue interspersed with energy-storing adipocytes (fat cells). Mainly used for fat storage.
http://en.wikipedia.org/wiki/Subcutaneous_tissue
Unfortunately, as you get older, your subcutaneous tissue begins to thin out.
http://www.innerbody.com/image_musfov/musc16-new.html

Lipids, collagen and elastin

Sebum

There are hundreds and hundreds of various moisturisers on the market all promising to be the best, to make you look wonderful but nature actually makes its' own skin moisturiser in the sebaceous glands.

Sebaceous glands secrete the oily, waxy substance called sebum (Latin, meaning fat or tallow) that is made of fat (lipids), wax, and the debris of dead fat-producing cells. In the glands, sebum is produced within specialized cells and is released as these cells burst; sebaceous glands are thus classified as holocrine glands. Seborrhoea is the name for the condition of greasy skin caused by excess sebum.
http://en.wikipedia.org/wiki/Sebaceous_gland

Collagen and elastin overview

Collagen and elastin are naturally occurring proteins that work together and are found in several parts of the body.

At the scientific level both are very complex and not fully understood. However, you can think of collagen as the rigid support for the skin, and internal tissues and the elastin as the stuff that makes them stretchable. Elastin provides flexibility, balancing the rigidity of collagen.

Elastin keeps the skin stretchy but firm, providing a snap-back reaction when tugged. Elastin returns the skin back to its regular shape after it's been extended. It keeps skin from sagging as it expands and contracts during normal activities.

Collagen

Collagen is a protein building block of bone, muscle, and all tissue throughout your body. It is the fibrous network holding all your parts and pieces together.

As the aging process begins (at approximately 27 years of age) various components that build bone, joint and muscle, cartilage, hair, and skin decline over the years. Collagen is one of the major building blocks in a group of body building components. Signs of collagen deficiency ever increase over the years.

Collagen is a major component of skin thickness. However it has been observed that with aging skin collagen decreases more rapidly than skin thickness – so say most but as with all science I did find a contradictory paper. In essence it said much depends on whether you tested facial or body skin. The debate goes on.

Variations in Facial Skin Thickness and Echogenicity with Site and Age.
"In our study skin thickness valuations of facial skin related to aging did not show a decreasing trend as on other areas. On the contrary significant increments in skin thickness values were observed at most of the assessed facial skin sites with 7% overall increase!!!!
Google - Acta Derm Venereol 1999;79:366±369.
Stefania Seidenari, Department of Dermatology, University of Modena, Via del Pozzo 71, IT-41100 Modena, Italy.

Therefore the word "collagen" has been hijacked by the skin cream market because a full face is a youthful looking face. Collagen depletes as we age. The collagen in skin creams cannot penetrate the outer layers of the skin. Even if collagen could get in and go under the skin – as is the case with injections – where the collagen just sits there for a while until it dissipates, the face is not stimulated to produce new collagen.

There are tons and tons of rubbish written about collagen on the internet and even I have had and do have problems trying to sort the wheat from the chaff.

To read more about this complex protein a good start would be
http://en.wikipedia.org/wiki/Collagen

How to build collagen

Sources of collagen

Collagen fibres are made from protein, and they are somewhat unusual in having large amounts of two amino acids, called hydroxy**lysine** and hydroxy**proline**.

Animal foods are the primary source of both amino acids.

Proline - egg whites appear to be an especially good source from amongst the animal foods and **wheat germ** amongst plant foods.

Lysine - lean meats, fish and low-fat dairy products would be especially concentrated sources.

One significant source from plant food category would be legumes (peas, beans, lentils, soy and particularly peanuts).
http://www.whfoods.com/genpage.php?

An easy way to boost the production of collagen production naturally in your body is to eat foods rich in antioxidants. Why? Antioxidants help control free radical damage to your cells. Healthy cell production gives collagen a better chance to rebuild.

Good food choices include carrots, tomatoes and green, leafy vegetables like Brussels sprouts and broccoli. Citrus fruits and melons (cantaloupe), and berries (blueberries, strawberries) are also excellent choices. Tuna fish and salmon, which are sources of omega-3 fatty acids, are also good for healthy skin.
http://www.streetarticles.com/anti-aging/how-to-build-collagen-in-skin-for-a-younger-look

Collagen supplements

Animal sources of collagen supplements commonly come from shark cartilage, young bovine (cows) cartilage, chicken comb, and a little bit of hog mixed in the group.

Plant sources of collagen supplements are found best in dark green vegetables. These followed by red fruits and vegetables with some dark fruits such as berries – blueberries, blackberries and currants.
http://www.joint-muscle-relief.com/how-to-build-collagen.html

Without question, the best vitamin you can take to boost not only antioxidant levels, but also increase collagen production is vitamin C. Citrus fruits and acids appear to be one of the best choices in the rebuilding of collagen in the skin.
http://www.streetarticles.com/anti-aging/how-to-build-collagen-in-skin-for-a-younger-look

Gelatin is an excellent source as it contains hydrolyzed collagen.

A preclinical study investigated the effects of oral ingestion of hydrolyzed collagen, along with vitamin C and glucosamine, suggested that the moisture content of skin, its viscoelastic properties, and smoothness benefit.
http://en.wikipedia.org/wiki/Hydrolyzed_collagen

Interesting collagen fact

Collagen cannot be absorbed through the skin; but collagen is now being used as a main ingredient for some cosmetic makeup. It is a complete and utter lie to suggest that it can, these products should be banned, hey maybe that will be my next campaign?!!

Collagen can be increased with exercise

Exercise increases collagen
"The stresses of exercise activate a particular molecular pathway that increases collagen," which leads to stronger connective tissues in the dermis, and thus, fewer wrinkles and younger-looking skin.
http://houseofverona.com/exercise-increases-collagen-ibuprofen-inhibits-this-effect/

An alternate way to increase collagen is to encourage the body's natural production and prevent collagen loss through diet and exercise.
http://www.wisegeek.com/how-do-i-increase-collagen.htm

As women get older, levels of collagen and other connective tissues diminish. Collagen is what keeps skin tight and youthful and doing resistance training can increase these collagen levels. Exercise helps flush out the body to keep skin healthy by increasing oxygen and nutrient supply to the skin cells. This helps maintain youthful appearance and reduces acne. The appearance of cellulite can also be reduced. The higher the fat level a woman has the more apparent the cellulite. Exercise helps by reducing overall fat levels and increasing collagen levels.
http://ezinearticles.com/?Benefits-of-Exercise-As-Women-Get-Older&id=5456682

Elastin

Elastin is our body's structural protein that gives elasticity to our tissues and organs. Elastin is found predominantly in the walls of our arteries, in our lungs, intestines, and skin, as well as in other elastic tissues. It functions in connective tissue in partnership with collagen. Whereas collagen provides rigidity, elastin is the protein which allows the connective tissues to stretch and then recoil to their original positions.

Imagine elastin within the body's connective tissue to act like a bunch of rubber bands that are tied together at a number of places. When the elastic bands are pulled, they will stretch, and when there is no longer a pull, they will return to their original relaxed state. You can't pull the elastin chain too far because the companion stiff collagen fibres in the connective tissue limit the stretching of the elastin fibres in the tissue

Elastin is considered by scientists to be a very tough and relatively stable protein because it has many internal linkages. Those linkages make elastin resistant to the normal breakdown which is normally characteristic of most other proteins

Since elastin is relatively stable, we do not need to make elastin throughout our lives. Normally the body stops making elastin once the body reaches maturity soon after puberty. A geneticist would say the same thing by stating that "the gene for elastin is turned off just after puberty." In other words, once the body has made its elastin, it will not make that protein any more.

The consequence of not being able to make any more elastin after we mature is aging begins!
http://www.wsf.org/medical/elastin.htm

Elastin, is a major cause of aging.
http://stretchmarkinstitute.com/18,elastin-in-normal-skin-and-damaged-how-does-it-work.html

What happens to elastin when the skin is overstretched?
Just like a rubber band that's been extended beyond its capacity, overstretched elastin cells are damaged beyond repair. Skin with ruined elastin is furrowed or saggy or pouchy.

Elastin is located under the surface, in the middle skin layer, the dermis. This is the skin's busy production centre, where intricate composition and maintenance is carried out 24-7. Here lie the connective tissue, small blood vessels, nerves and cells that replicate the major skin component, collagen.

Thickness of Aging Skin

In fact, among dermatological researchers there is great controversy about the effects of aging on the thickness of skin strata.
/www.alluredbooks.com/sample_pages/a_derm_view_ch35.pdf

Vitamin C is good for skin regeneration

These results will be of great relevance to the cosmetics industry. Free radicals are associated with premature skin aging, and antioxidants, such as vitamin C, are known to counter these highly damaging compounds. This new evidence suggest that, in addition to 'mopping up' free radicals, vitamin C can help remove the DNA damage they form, if they get past the cell's defences.
http://www.science20.com/news_articles/vitamin_c_linked_human_skin_regeneration

Toxicity of vitamins

When the body recognizes that the intake of water soluble vitamins exceeds daily needs, the elimination process becomes more efficient and the excess is voided from the body in the urine. With fat soluble vitamins there is more danger. Fat soluble vitamins are not as quickly eliminated from the body, but rather are stored in fat tissues and in various organs throughout the body.

You can overdose on any vitamin supplement if you take it long enough and in high enough doses. Since only the fat-soluble vitamins---A, D, E and K---are stored in your body in greater-than-needed amounts, they are the ones mostly like to reach toxic levels. Vitamin D has the potential to be more toxic than any other vitamin. Vitamin E toxicity, on the other hand, is uncommon, and when it does occur, it is less serious than toxicity from vitamins A, D and K.
http://www.livestrong.com/article/22298-vitamin-toxicity-symptoms/

Chapter 4

The alternatives

Natural - other face exercise
(non "hands free" methods)
Topical treatments - creams
Non-invasive - gadgets
Invasive procedures - needles & knives

MISINFORMATION FACTS
Read the facts and then skip the chapter if you like

Skin creams containing collagen cannot work
as they cannot penetrate the outer layers of the skin
therefore collagen must be injected
(normally harvested from young beef cattle)

The body stops producing elastin at puberty!
It is impossible to stimulate natural production of elastin
except with HGH (which is very dangerous)
THE TRUTH ABOUT HUMAN GROWTH HORMONE
http://www.therealessentials.com/hgh1.html

BOTOX® can travel to the brain and surrounding tissues
Needles and knives do and can kill you.
BOTOX® was only legal FDA approved April 12 2002
http://en.wikipedia.org/wiki/Botulinum_toxin

The best way to prevent premature aging is facial exercise,
preferably with Fitface "hands-free" facial toning.

You have the freedom of choice

To either, spend 10 minutes every other day facial toning with

Fitface - Nature's beauty spa
to have glowing, great looking healthy skin
and
rejuvenate your face,
to prevent wrinkles from forming in the first place
or

Use a cream or serum
But you will only be treating the surface

Inject something under healthy skin,
for a short term result
which in the long-term does more harm than good.

A neurotoxin will stop dynamic wrinkles
But nature responds by using other muscles
Hence more wrinkles

A filler will "plump up" and out the skin
But nature responds by stretching the skin
Over time this weakens the skin's natural tissue structures.
Thus, the skin thins and loses its elasticity
Hence more filler are required sooner,
to cure the self inflicted damage from needles!
Creating a vicious circle that you are dependent on for life!
A merry-go-round of addiction to injections
until you are all "puffed up" like a chipmunk!

Then
More injections - hence more dependency on needles!

Then, cosmetic surgery, a facelift to pull up the sagging face,
shorten muscles and insert implants
Resulting in dependency on facelifts!

Why start? It's insanity!

Start Fitface Today
To
Naturally build collagen and tone all over the face.
You know it makes sense!

Personal note

I cannot understand why facial exercises are not a part of everyday life as they are in China. Not solely for cosmetic purposes or even just eyesight, but also for hearing, taste and smell too. To me it is madness not to exercise the face. There may even be another reason for men; hair growth (and women for that matter too). A full head of healthy-looking hair is all part of a youthful, fresh healthy vital look. (Check out Jack Lalanne on You Tube at 96!!)

I can only think that some people might still believe the outdated, outlandish idea that facial exercise causes wrinkles. Why would it? How could it? Does it? No, of course not! The opposite is true; exercise removes wrinkles (stuck in a groove). By lack of movement.

Are you still sceptical? Then do, take a look at other facial exercise guru's and ask yourself "Are they disfigured by hundreds of wrinkles?" Of course not; facial exercise does not make wrinkles but prevents static wrinkles from forming. The truth is that these women look as good (if not even better and certainly far softer and more natural looking) than the rich and famous celebrities of the same age that have had to resort to needles and or knives.

The 50 sexiest women over 50
http://www.zimbio.com/The+50+Sexiest+Women+Over+50
The 50 most beautiful women over 50
h/www.stylebistro.com/The+50+Most+Beautiful+Women+Over+50

A new phenomenon is that they really are all beginning to look the same – odd!

Think about facial exercise logically. Stop listening to old-fashioned ideas that you once believed that were reported by the media beauty machine. They all want to sell you their solution advertised by a model or endorsed by a celebrity (who was paid millions) and both were assisted by Adobe® Photoshop® to sell you an unobtainable dream.

Fitface is virtually free; it does not cost a fortune. Fitface always puts health before beauty. There is no risk, no pain, no swelling, no bruising, no lumps, no scaring, no physiological addition such as **Wrinklerexia** or dependency, no allergic reaction, and no migration to the brain, no complications, no disfigurements, no deformities, and no deaths. The results in the short term are not as dramatic as surgery but in the long-term I can guarantee you will not look like a freak causing you acute distress.

Facial exercise methods

The main difference between Fitface and the other facial exercise methods is that I am the only facial exercise guru who believes in the "hands free" method. Obviously, I think my way is best, and I am sure the others think that their way is best. My view is that because we cannot naturally reproduce any elastin to make the skin stretchy after puberty, why would one risk putting any pressure on the face that is unnecessary? Fitface exercise never stretches the skin beyond that which it can do naturally.

I am so anti needles and knives that I would prefer anyone to use any form of facial exercise from almost any of my competitors (with the exception of one) rather than resort to the extremes of needles or knives. Yes, I am old-fashioned and do think that is dishonest to promote something that you do not yourself believe in. Practice what you preach.

Without naming names (or giving you the YouTube link to one of the most famous facial exercise gurus) I would like to point out that she has bravely admitted publicly - on national TV - that she has had "work done" some years ago for a nasal medical problem! This is an admission of **cosmetic surgery**; which is fair enough but perhaps not for someone who advocates facial exercise after the fact. I would further add that in my opinion, judging from how she looks; that recently she has had some more "nasal problems" as facial exercises do not give you the wind tunnel lift!

What she does is her business but I do feel that it is misleading, something that I normally associate with the cosmeceutical and pharmaceutical companies. Not with face and neck aficionados. *Somehow, "it's just not cricket." Worse it denigrates facial exercises.*

There is one book on the subject of face and a neck exercise that has latched on to the exercise buzz word "isometric" which is fine. Unfortunately the way this lady explains how an isometric exercise works is incorrect. I would write and explain it to her but perhaps it was just an error, as I do not think it was in anyway an attempt to mislead the public. It's a shame as she was my favourite but I think she means well but may be misinformed or have misunderstood her research. Watch out, check it for yourself.

Topical treatments

Creams

Over the counter creams

An ordinary simple (preferably pH balanced) moisturising creams is all you need. They all act as a barrier and trap water and natural emollients produced by your skin from being lost.

Regrettably the over-the-counter anti-aging creams don't do what they say on the box. There are no LAWS in place to ensure that it should, in today's world we take the information at face value. Society believes that "the more you pay the better the product works" knowing that, the brand manager prices the product to suit the pockets of the clients perceptions. Therefore, contrary to most marketing mixes; the more expensive the more demand, and to increase demand limits supply. It works for the huge French brands.

If the cream could do what they imply they can, then most of the products would need a prescription! The same goes for serums, which are just an even fancier way of exploiting the fountain of youth market.

In the medical world, clinically proven means that a product has some positive action on some biological function and this has been demonstrated by well-controlled clinical studies by reputable researchers. However, in the cosmetic industry, this term can mean anything. Many products that have never been tested in any clinical study are deemed clinically proven. Most commonly, this means that some component of the cosmetic product has been shown in some study, somewhere, sometime, to have had some biological action. For example: a product may contain vitamin C and since vitamin C has been clinically proven to be a necessary vitamin, this somehow means that the cosmetic product is clinically proven **without trials of that cream**.

When I first began researching I thought a clinical trial was an excellent way to see if a product worked but I soon found out it was not all that it was cracked up to be, especially not for cosmetic products. For example: I read a very positive test result for a cream. However, when I delved deeper into the report I read that the trial was conducted in Africa on very mature women with weather beaten skin. It is therefore, hardly surprising that the product showed such a good result but legally that information need not be disclosed. Moreover, to clarify my findings I discussed the issue with a good friend of mine who lives in California and has a company that writes clinical medical trials. She confirmed my suspicious.

Prescribed cosmetic creams *(I am not discussing ointments for medical reasons)*

I am not anti creams to hydrate externally and moisturise the outer layers of the skin, they are great superficially but then can do nothing for the muscles or build your collagen regardless of the claims. Collagen molecules are just simply too big to penetrate the external layers! That's why they are injected. Ask, inquire, and know exactly what you are being sold. Why not ask to see the clinical trials the test results? You are not being obstreperous, merely you are an individual with a critical thought processes.

Please do not misunderstand me; prescribed skin creams are excellent for medical conditions. Also some cosmetic skin creams for example, to fade 'age spots' but here I am discussing expensive anti-aging lotions and potions; such as **Creme de la Mer.**

I had never heard of Crème de la Mer but I asked a friend of mine what she would buy if she had the money and she said Creme de la Mer because Kylie uses it! I thought I would investigate and this is what I found.

Creme de la Mer (Estee Lauder) is a fermentation product that was invented by a German rocket scientist, Max Huber, but it is basically a throwback to European peasant therapies. It is a combination of kelp, alfalfa, sunflowers, eucalyptus, vitamins and minerals which is fermented for five months while enzymes break down the plants into small fragments.

The source of the idea is from European peasants who would use fermented plants (often the silage used for cow feed) to put on wounds. The fermenting plants become very warm and a handful of the plants or silage would be put on wounds and held in place with a bandage. There is no proof that these methods actually increase skin repair but the heat from the fermenting plants would increase blood flow to the injured skin and probably increase healing.
http://www.skinbiology.com/expensiveskincreams.html
It costs £530 a pot - but the ingredients cost just £25... the brow-furrowing truth about the stars' favourite wrinkle cream, Crème de la Mer
http://www.dailymail.co.uk/femail/beauty/article-1242978/Cr-la-Mer--It-costs-530-pot--ingredients-cost-just-25--brow-furrowing-truth-stars-favourite-wrinkle-cream.html#ixzz1rqLHYsiN

Skincare as we age
The beauty industry flouts the words collagen and elastin as ingredient in many anti aging creams. This is because colllagen **and elastin** are the skin proteins responsible for elasticity, tone and texture. Glycosoaminoglycans (GAG's or mucopolysaccharides) and proteoglycans hold water in the skin) and are the true skin moisturisers. In contrast, cosmetic moisturizers cover the skin with a water impermeable barrier such

as petrolatum or heavy oil. This artificially slows the loss of moisture from the skin and gives the skin a temporary appearance of plumpness and fullness.
http://www.skinbiology.com/skinhealth&aging.html

Post menopausal
(A nightmare, I have aged 10 years in 4)!

I have on occasion had to resort to a thicker moisturiser than my normal E45 moisturising lotion (not available in the USA). For my American friends I often take some over. It's Dermatological, Perfume Free Hypoallergenic and says is soothes, softens and relieves dry and sensitive skin on the bottle. I'm not keen on the thicker E45 cream, for me it's too thick, a bit like Nivea cream. I do like Flexitol Intense Hydrating Lotion – it does say, "Clinically proven to increase skin hydration" which I take with a pinch of salt. I first came across Flexitol in the States as a heel balm and it was/is miraculous so when I searched for something with more punch I thought I would try it. They also make Flexitol Very Dry Skin Cream but I'm not so keen on that.

Elastin

Elastin and collagen are partners, and the fibres that interlace purposefully. They create the combination of plasticity and tautness that makes up normal skin. Sudden increases in growth or/and weight caused after puberty such as pregnancy, fat gain or muscle gain, and the corresponding changes in hormone levels, wreak havoc upon skin where the stretching is greatest. Collagen production gets disrupted. And Elastin loses its function. With the two main constituents malfunctioning, the dermis is likely to tear. These tears become visible in the surface skin layer, the epidermis, which has been considerably thinned by the stretching an example of which in the case of pregnancy are called stretch marks.

What happens to elastin when the skin is overstretched?

Just like a rubber band that's been extended beyond its capacity, overstretched elastin cells can be damaged beyond repair. Skin with ruined elastin is furrowed, saggy or pouchy. Elastin is located under the surface, in the middle skin layer, the dermis. This is the skin's busy production centre, where intricate composition and maintenance is carried out 24-7. Here lie the connective tissue, small blood vessels, nerves and cells that replicate the major skin component, collagen.

Is there a way to add new elastin into the face?

My research says **no**. However there is so much elastin written/advertised and said to be in cosmetic products that I have tried to go with the flow (against my better judgement) and written as if there was the remotest chance that it could be sourced and then either injected or put in a cream. I am having a really hard time writing that and moreover – if injected, why and how would an animal source integrate within in human skin? The more seriously I contemplate the matter the more ludicrous it becomes but I will press on disregarding my intelligent mindset.

There are anti-stretch mark lotions and creams that have collagen and elastin added. The promoters of these products make it all sound so easy: just rub the cream in and your skin will become perfect. But, that's just pie in the sky.

The trouble with these tonics is that the additives so needed to build up new skin aren't likely to penetrate into the dermis, where all skin production takes place. The molecules of collagen and elastin are too big to get through. Another concern is the origin of the collagen is harvested from cattle and birds, and the medical community worries that this is a pathway for Mad Cow disease or swine flu.

Meanwhile, the promoter of a lotion or serum that's packed with collagen must specify the importance of vigorous massage to help open pores to let it in. If massage isn't part of the instruction, then the advertising is really quite false. There's only the slimmest of slim chance that prior rubbing will work, but by directing the buyer to deeply massage before applying the serum, at least the promoter is in some way attempting to overcome the fact of non-absorption.

Accordingly, practitioners of laser therapy and micro-dermabrasion must firmly instruct their patients to apply lotions between treatments. The procedures stimulate natural collagen production and breaks down corneocytes, the impermeable coating of the **dermis**.

Wouldn't it be great if elastin could replicate! Imagine not needing a tummy tuck, or the tightening of saggy breasts. Imagine watching your tummy get right back to taut, before your baby's first feeding. And imagine your breasts staying plump and firm always, just like they were when full of milk. Keep working on it, venerable white coats. We're waiting with baited breath!
http://stretchmarkinstitute.com/18,elastin-in-normal-skin-and-damaged-how-does-it-work.html

Collagen

Although collagen cannot be absorbed through the skin, collagen is now being used as a main ingredient for some cosmetic makeup. Amazing!
http://en.wikipedia.org/wiki/Collagen

Creams and serums feel great but none of them can lift sagging jowls the way face exercises can and collagen cannot even get in let alone work!

The internet has made it far easier for me to do research but even so, sadly there is so much rubbish out there trying to make you buy something; (especially any anti-aging product - chiefly creams) that scientific research is cluttered by misleading advertisements making it almost impossible to source the truth. There is so much "clutter," an abundance of misinformation about products and the finding that real useful information is either camouflaged or hidden.

I have delved into many research papers that are normally only available to the medical profession (whom hold expensive licences and therefore are privy to the inner sanctum of information) and found some alarming results. Without sounding too dramatic some of the reports that I have managed to see are shocking. The executives that head these companies should be ashamed of themselves for making **billions of pounds KNOWING the product DOES NOT WORK.** They have the complete proof from the clinical trials that proves conclusively that a product is not effective but they go ahead and market it anyway. The marketing mix works; -.throw in some hope (LOADS - BY THE BUCKET FULL – aimed at the 40+market) toss in the words "looking younger or more beautiful" add in a celebrity endorsement, sprinkle with Adobe® Photoshop®, place into great packaging and add an expensive price tag and "Bob's your uncle" you have a winner.

Clinical trials on over- the-counter cosmetics must prove that the product is safe but that is all – NOTHING MORE. They do not have to prove the product works or works for the condition that it is being sold for as discussed earlier.

Celebrities are mainly singers or actors (what do they know about skincare??? They employ people who do know)! But they supplement and/or enhance their incomes/fame by endorsing various products in the knowledge that their fans will buy them but it was not what made them famous. On the other hand "models" become famous because what they advertise sells; it is an honest living, they are paid to sell product. I am not knocking either, but enjoy looking at the adverts for what they are – fantasy.
http://www.skinbiology.com/expensiveskincreams.html

Tretinoin aka (Retin-A, Avita, Renova)
I put this section is as a surprise for DW in SC - can't help myself sometimes!

Tretinoin is the acid form of vitamin A to treat acne and reduce oiliness in the skin. For which my research seems to suggest that it works, but for purely cosmetic benefits, then, umm it's far more sketchy.

Note:
Many people confuse retinol with Retin-A (tretinoin). Retinol and retinoic acid (tretinoin) are related but distinctly different. Retinol, retinal and retinyl palmitate, do not have the same effect on the skin as tretinoin/retinoic acid. They first need to be converted by special enzymes into the active metabolite, retinoic acid. Unfortunately, the conversion rate is low and varies among individuals. The other problem is that **when retinols are exposed to air, they can become oxidized and degraded.** There are some companies that have produced retinol formulas that are more stabilized.

Side effects of Retin-A

The effect of increased skin cell turnover can be irritation and flaking. For this reason, many people stop using Retin-A after a couple of days to weeks, then think that it didn't work. It is important to realize that Retin-A is very effective for whiteheads and blackheads, but it may take 6-9 weeks to see a noticeable difference. It takes at least 6 months to see a noticeable difference in wrinkles. The best benefit is seen if Retin-A is used for at least a year.

Does it work? *(I know Dianne is thinking that!)*

Well, I've not use it. Okay, I do get the odd pimple/spot/zit if I really down the sweets/candies for a couple of days. But although I do binge - as a rule I normally don't. So I only have a couple of old acne scars from smallpox which I contracted at 39 years old (Yes, I did nearly die from it)!

I put it to her this way almost verbatim (save grammar adjustments).

Don't touch Tretonion with a barge pole. Think logically about it! Your skin is there to protect you and then you throw on a mild acid -Tretonion. The mind boggles!

What do you think the skin thinks???

The skin thinks: "It's an invader! An invader, help! "Need to protect" ...panic!!!

Yes, they (serious /prescription skin creams) can help for a while BUT CANNOT POSSIBLY alter the skins' natural biology to build anything up, they can only destroy things such as pigment, age spots and fade scars.

I guess they may work but at what cost? (I would love to hear) but I do worry that then, (as with the test results on lipids) that the skin will stop producing its natural "stuff".
http://en.wikipedia.org/wiki/Tretinoin
http://dermatology.about.com/cs/topicals/a/tretinoin.htm
http://bestofbothworldsaz.com/2010/10/18/the-truth-about-tretinoin-retin-a/
http://bestofbothworldsaz.com/2010/10/18/the-truth-about-tretinoin-retin-a/

In my search for the ultimate skin care cream I came across this article and thought it was worth highlighting. It makes you understand how clever Mother Nature is:

Skin lipid replacement products

Are very expensive skin creams worth the price?

Extract: One approach to skin repair was to coat the skin with a mixture of lipids that closely approximately natural skin lipids (fats). When applied to dry and cracking skin, this method produced very rapid (within 2 hours) and striking changes in water loss across the skin barrier and this was called "skin repair." The problem with this method was that the added lipids caused a later inhibition of the skin's natural lipid production in a process called in biochemical terms "feedback inhibition." The ultimate result is that the shutting down of the skin's lipid biosynthesis leads to a skin state that is worse than before the application of the lipids.
http://www.skinbiology.com/expensiveskincreams.html

Mother Nature can be very clever *(it is a shame to see the new 2012 UK Tampax advert which is so vilifying towards her - without whom we/reproduction would not exist)* and decided that there was no need to produce natural emollients, wisely turning her resources to producing something else! The good news is that if you stop using the product, after 28 days Mother Nature thinks um, better start production again. The problem is that one thinks "the cream worked" my skin looks dreadful when I stop using it - before giving nature a chance to kick back in again.

Facial Exercises are a must for anyone who has tried an anti-aging cream and has been disappointed.

Non invasive treatments
Gadgets & treatments

The list is too long to cover them all in any detail, after all this book is supposed to be about the exercises and I haven't even started yet!

Exfoliating scrubbers, facial brushes

There are hundreds of new products to temp you and me. I've tried many in the vain hope of finding something useful, even a scrubber because at my age (56), I do now believe in very GENTLE exfoliation. Post menopausal skin sheds less often and sometime I need a little help. I've tried all sorts but haven't found anything more successful than a £1 exfoliating glove. I try not overdo it as I understand that I will lose essential lipids and emollients in the underneath layers.

I tried using the glove with a mild face cream but found that all a little messy. Instead I cut the fingers off and cut the hand portion into pieces. Then using just one finger dipped it in my good old standby E45 lotion and made gentle small circular motions to remove the flakes. I certainly do have more now that I am old, yes despite my exercises.

I also bought a softer option, a rotating brush with different heads but I found that both messy and noisy, so I'm back to the glove, especially as I get a little dry skin near the corner of my eye and which irritates me but it is easily removed with a finger.

Electric muscle stimulating machines

Electrical muscle stimulation (EMS) uses a mild electrical current to exercise your muscles move. An electrical current passes through the skin to the nerves in that area, causing the muscle to expand and contract. but the action is involuntary muscle contraction and not a voluntary movement as with facial exercise. This confuses the body as it is not a natural process. Somewhere I read that they do not work very well because they stimulate a different neurological pathway to the brain.

I did like the idea of a face EMS machine and I did try a few. They felt as if they were working but somehow just not as well as doing it yourself perhaps it's because the body can't be fooled. Perhaps it's because when you exercise the face you exercise more than just the muscles?

I'm not sure. I don't think they do any harm because ultimately they do the same thing as Fitface, but it's just not natural.

What I am not so sure about is how "hands free" some of them are. I think used as instructed they are fine but open a few I have seen are open to pressure abuse, which although elastin is very durable may not be used to the combination of electrical stimulus and exercise. *So for me, I'm sticking with Fitface.*

Photon, Ultrasound and Galvanic devices

Photon (light) therapy

There was so much positive press about photon therapy and therefore, the beauty industry was very excited about the possible implications. However, it is still early days.

Light therapy

Intense Pulsed Light (IPL) and Light-Emitting Diode (LED) light therapies have been known to increase the production of natural collagen as well as the level of blood circulation. Light therapy comes in many different shapes and sizes, and primarily is based on the concept of multiple wavelengths of light energy being sent through the skin creating heat in the dermis that stimulates cellular activity.

Deep photon infrared LED light

In the laboratory, Whelan and his team have shown that skin and muscle cells, grown in cultures and exposed to the LED infrared light, grow 150 to 200 percent faster than ground control cultures not stimulated by the light. Scientists are trying to learn how cells

convert light into energy, and identify which wavelengths of light are most effective at stimulating growth in different kinds of cells.
http://www.budwigcenter.com/photon-infrared-therapy.php

There are many commercial and home devices on the market claiming all sorts of results. All the websites selling these devices seem to make sense. In a nut shell most explain that they heat under the skin which damages the skin **which can** stimulate the cells and cause growth and repair

The Photon Beauty Device, designed for facial beautification, uses natural light waves, which are transmitted by LEDs into the skin. The light activates photoreceptors in skin cells, producing energy for absorption by skin components, to beautify your complexion.

Studies show that light enters the body as photons (energy) and is absorbed by the photoreceptors within cells. Massaging with the Photon Beauty balances skin tone and enhances circulation. Light is known **for helping with some** beauty problems, for instance, inhibiting the formation of melanin pigment, fighting acne and dermatitis, and improving the look of pockmarks, scars and wrinkles.
www.ib3health.com/products/PhotonBeauty/PhotonBeautyIndex.shtml

They all sound very impressive, and all the sales literature makes you want to sit up and listen. It all sounds highly technical, medical and proves they work! I so wanted to find something that really worked. I thought it would make a great addition to my book, perhaps packaged with the book as a Christmas gift? I enthusiastically ploughed through all the information I could get my hands on, studied endlessly websites and read product literature about photon therapy and ultrasound for facial rejuvenation as they are often sold by the same companies or come together in a hand-held unit. The ultrasonic part in the middle with LED lights around the edge. At the time I thought I was an expert, well very informed by all the narrative I had received from the manufacturers of professional machines. I was so impressed by the entire bumph that I ordered a few samples of the home devices for experimentation.

After trying them all; I came to the sad conclusion that nothing worked. Perhaps they were not strong enough because of making them safe for the home market? Although with one of the photon devices I did get the machine with the largest number of LED's (light-emitting diodes) that I thought was in the "reasonably priced" bracket. It had hundreds (I'm not sure exactly how many, it sits in a drawer, and I can't count them all). Looking for an answer for inclusion in this book, I turned to the instruction manual and read the penultimate phrase "The photon device **may** activate the human cell at 5 times the rate……etc. It's all down to the word **may** which means there are no guarantees. Therefore, I must now conclude that sales and results are based on hope.

There were three light settings a red, a blue and a combination of the two. I had used the red setting on the pulse mode daily to treat my red skin patches that I get whenever I eat certain foods. Yes I know, I should cut them out entirely but being a vegetarian I would be left with less choice, so I put up with it. Anyway, the device did nothing to clear the condition in the first week. Concerned that they had not disappeared, I stopped eating spicy foods, processed foods, tomatoes, cheese and oranges – my trigger foods. But, the next week I looked even worse than the week before! I was getting very anxious but pressed on in the vain hope that perhaps I needed to look worse before I looked better as is the purported case with laser. Very worried I only managed to hang in there one more week. I really looked bad, so I stopped.

Perhaps I should try the device again, perhaps I should try all the other machines again, perhaps I didn't give them long enough but now perhaps I know too much too. For example, if I read the sales paraphernalia and it says something that I know to be incorrect like "**it stimulates elastin growth**" – which I know to be IMPOSSIBLE, therefore, I immediately shut down and whatever else is written I consider to be rubbish.

There is a fairly new device on the market called Fine Light Mask by Innovate Photonices. It looked interesting until I read how it stimulated elastin, so once again my hopes were dashed.
http://fine-light.co.uk/how-led-light-therapy-works.html

Ultrasound

Works by sending sound waves through the skin to stimulate the cells; but once again, the home device I tried did nothing for me.

Having since read this article, I am not surprised that it didn't work for me:
An extract from a clinical trial dated 2007:
Selective transcutaneous delivery of energy to porcine (pig) soft tissues using Intense Ultrasound (IUS).
CONCLUSION: This study demonstrates the response of porcine tissue to various energy dose levels of Intense Ultrasound. Further study, especially on human facial tissue, is necessary in order to understand the utility of this modality in treating the aging face and potentially, other cosmetic applications."

Such articles make me think "What, that was only 5 years ago?! I thought they knew already it worked before putting it on the market for sale but obviously not!"

Ultrasonic massager

Ultrasonic waves can permeate into deep tissues, radiating heat to stimulate and invigorate; the micro-vibration stimulate cells, sparking re-growth and an accelerated recovery effect.

I do think it would help aid the passage of a cream through the epidermis. However, I have not tried it, as I am not a believer in "creams"

Galvanic treatment

Galvanic treatment refers to skin treatment using galvanic ions. A galvanic massager works by boosting the absorption of water soluble skin care nutrients deep into the skin using galvanic ions. The two forces (+ positive and - negative) pull together like a magnet and push the product into the deeper layers of the skin (the dermis). (+)Positive ions aid in the removal of toxins and impurities. (-)Negative ions encourage the transport of beneficial nutrients which deliver re-energizing results.

The product for home use is sold with a gel, and I think that the results of the treatment have more to do with the gel used than the device itself. However, the literature sort of implies that anyway.

At the spa it would probably be called a micro-current toning anti-aging facial. They became all the rage several years ago after being featured on Oprah for its dramatic anti-aging benefits.

D. Tsoklis, an expert on the subject, also explains: *"Micro-current is the reproduction of your own biological current. As we age, this current, which sends messages from the brain to the muscles via the spinal cord, does not send those messages properly."*

- Of those that participated in the study, 52.4% experienced positive changes in the UV spots (caused by sun/ UV damage) appearing on their face; showing as much as 46.1% improvement, or reduction in UV spots. The photos reveal impressive and consistent trends in tissue repair.
- Forty-three percent of participants experienced a reduction in wrinkles; 14.3% was the greatest wrinkle reduction on measure in this minimal four session study.
http://www.thequantumalliance.com/eternale/science/

Skin analysing machines

I tried a couple of inexpensive home ones and was disappointed to find that there was no consistency with the reading, so I gave up.

I certainly did like the look of a professional skin analyzing machine that cost thousands. I hoped that put in the right hands of an experienced doctor, and after a succession of procedures real positive results could be achieved. I do feel that this is the first step in seeking appropriate and accurate treatment of any kind. Without a dermatologist/doctor knowing precisely what and where problem is on your face. How can a doctor correctly offer a solution? Especially as in one study it was found that as much as 30% of the inconsequential facial muscles were incapable of working correctly because of inappropriate attachments into other muscles or they were simply missing! Hence, the needs for a precise diagnosis of the tissues of your face as 1 in 3 faces are structurally different.

Even so, what good is analyzing the skin, i.e. knowing what the exact problems are, if you cannot do anything to solve the problem?

Lasers

There is a new hand held home laser on the market. It's expensive, but compared to trips to the spa it might be the answer for some. From what I have read it is my understanding that there are two drawbacks:
- Firstly, the size of the area that is targeted
- Secondly, home devices are super safe and therefore the power they exhibit is normally insufficient to be effectual

Professional laser treatments

They all have fancy names, and all promise to do all sorts of things; mainly rejuvenation. Many claim that they can stimulate elastin growth but my research informs me that there is nothing that can do that. Elastin cannot be stimulated to grow past puberty without adding Growth Hormone, which is very dangerous in my opinion because of the correlation with cancer. (HGH stimulates growth, i.e. multiplication of cells and cancer is out of control growth). Therefore, whatever else a clinic or spa says about their laser treatments I take with "a pinch of salt" even though they may have other great benefits such as for stimulating collagen growth and circulation. Which facial exercise does anyway!

- However, I have heard that in the right hands pigmentation marks such as liver spots/sun damage and acne lesions can be significantly reduced.

- My only experience was about 10 years ago. I had a laser treatment for red veins and to cut a long story short I looked shocking afterwards, like I had massively bad sunburn. Months and months passed before I healed, so unfortunately once bitten twice shy.

- I still do believe that something will come along which is great and I do hope that professional services are improving.

Resurfacing

A chemical peel is exactly what its name implies; acid on the face to burn off the skin. Yuk! Chemical peels are used to lift off the dead upper layers of your skin and are popular because they offer almost immediate results. but sadly don't last because we are constantly making new skin and sloughing it off.

I am also anti laser resurfacing. Micro-abrasion or acid/chemical peels. For me they are all far too hash for the skin, they send your face into "panic mode" as the body desperately tries to repair the self-inflicted damage, worse t hey and don't last. The skin was not designed to tolerate that much abuse, hence a red face as the body desperately fights to repair the self-inflicted damage. *With exercise you get a "glow," not a bright red face crying out in pain!*

Fractional laser skin resurfacing works by splitting the laser's light into tiny beams that are each about one-tenth the size of a hair shaft. The light penetrates the skin to a controlled depth, where its heat vaporizes the targeted cells, while leaving the tiny areas around each tiny beam of light untouched. Only about 20 to 30 percent of the targeted area is actually treated, yet the entire area benefits from the process and eventually becomes rejuvenated. And because less skin is actually damaged by the laser, the recovery time is generally shorter than with non-fractional CO_2 lasers.

I personally believe that resurfacing is too destructive for the skin. I feel that gentle exfoliation is quite hash enough to remove dead cells even for mature skin.

Mesotherapy

There are two types of mesotherapy:
- Invasive – needles, a few or many tiny, tiny ones
- Non invasive – electric pulses

Mesotherapy injections drive natural substances (no drugs) - such as a multivitamin blend or artichoke extract - four to six millimetres below the epidermis. Apparently, to use the body's own systems to repair and rebuild to improve skin's texture and tone.

There are different mesotherapy guns to inject between eight and 16 minuscule shots (each roughly 0.02 ccs of liquid, or one fifth the size of a raindrop) of a customized solution into the skin.

So far, there's just one peer-reviewed study addressing facial mesotherapy. "It probably does promote some anti-ageing," says David J. Goldberg, MD, a clinical professor of dermatology at NYC's Mount Sinai School of Medicine and co author of the only published research on the treatment. "However, without clinical results, it's really medi-spa hype at this point." His research, which appeared in the journal Dermatologic Surgery, examined 10 subjects who underwent four sessions of vitamin mesotherapy. After six months, "there was no statistically significant improvement," Goldberg says, "but we did see some microscopic evidence of new collagen formation."

With the non invasive procedure a wand is passed over the face and the muscles twitch. I had not tried the procedure but apparently the skin glows – for me just like it does after exercise. So why bother?

Invasive procedures
The slippery slope of dependency

If one starts with needles be it only beginning with mesotherapy, as young as 22 years old it really is a slippery slope downwards. At present rates of dissatisfaction with every decreasing satisfaction with the way you looked you would probably be having your first facelift at 35 and the next at age 42. By the time you are 50 you will need another one with implants along the way. Some celebrities have done just that, and we've all seen what a state they look, like freaks but it begins in all innocence. All too quickly it goes from Lasers to BOTOX®, to fillers, to implants, to facelifts to looking freaky. You cannot beat the age clock. Time and aging will eventually outlast any facelift result no matter how it is done.

If you must start with needles or knives, **please delay the start** until later, because then, at least you may only have one or two facelifts before (hopefully) you really don't care anymore as other health issues will have superseded the beauty criteria.

Fitface face exercises can make you glow with toned radiant good looks along the way, and by the time you are mature you may have been convinced that Fitface is the only way to go.

Misleading and Inappropriate use of medical terms

Unfortunately, in order to lessen the fear of needles, the risk of infection and complications occurring from invasive procedures the word "non" has been hijacked and put before the word invasive to make non-invasive procedures. **This is incorrect and should not be permitted by the medical profession.** As any procedure involving a needle for an injection will puncture the skin and therefore, should be correctly termed invasive.
http://www.nygplasticsurgery.com/medical-spa/

It seems that anyone can mislead the public if they choose to; there may be rules in place, but they are not adhered to. Here in the UK, we have the Advertising Standards Authority and one can write in to complain, but surely they should be policing the industry? Not us the public! The bigger problem is that when one company flouts the rules and gets away with it the whole industry follows suit (to pull the wool over the eyes of the unsuspecting public).
http://www.asa.org.uk/

It was hailed as an enormous victory when Member of Parliament Jo Swinson stood up against L'Oreal, she was opposed to the adverts for anti-wrinkle cream featuring actress Rachel Weisz. The adverts were banned (following her complaint), and the advert for Revitalift repair, was judged by the Advertising Standards Authority to have "misleadingly exaggerated" the product after Weisz's skin was retouched.

Previously, Swinson has successfully made complaints against a Lancome advert featuring Julia Roberts and a Maybelline advert featuring the supermodel Christy Turlington. **The Huffington Post**

UK Dina Rickman First Posted: 1/02/2012. But my point is that they should not have been allowed to "air" in the first place!

Flab jab by syringe

It's a controversial treatment, the "thin injection" or "lipodissolve" whereby the patient is given injections of tiny quantities of a fat-burning medication that can cause jowls and chubby chins to simply melt away. There were major problems with lumps and swelling with Lipostabil in the USA and there was a warning put out against it and the MHRA banned advertising for it. Now Bayer has produced a substance known as ATX-101 with the active ingredient being deoxycholate. It is undergoing trials and may be available in Europe by 2012. *My advice is, why be a human guinea pig? It is utter madness to even contemplate such tom foolery.*

Injectables by needle

There are two types of products administered by injection to help to remedy the signs of aging in the short term.

Dermal neurotoxins like the popular BOTOX® type treatments or **Dermal fillers** (soft tissue filling agents), like injectable collagen, fat or hyaluronic acid

The two types of fillers are generally divided into two broad categories: those which are used to treat dynamic wrinkles and those intended to reduce or eliminate the appearance of static wrinkles.

Dynamic wrinkles appear as a result of facial expression, such as smiling or frowning to stop any movement these muscles are treated with a neurotoxin.

Static wrinkles are lines, which occur as a result of sagging or loss of elasticity and moisture retention are treated with fillers.

Neurotoxins

BOTOX® is the product of choice, a nerve agent that paralyzes nerves. BOTOX® acts as a neuromuscular blocker when injected into the muscle. It works at the nerve endings and binds with them to block the nerve signal to the muscle. **It effectively filters the brain signals and the muscles do contract.** Therefore they artificially remain relaxed and frown lines, crow's feet, and other dynamic wrinkles cannot be formed and therefore, do not appear on the face.

What are the side effects of BOTOX®?

The most common side effect of BOTOX® injections are short-term pain, temporary swelling, bruising and in the long-term more wrinkles!!!!

"Over the past 15 years, BOTOX® has been embraced by thousands of women - the market in the **"forehead freezing drug"** is worth almost **£18 million** in the UK alone. However, it seems that one of its least-known **side-effects was** that if you use it a lot, or have it injected by an inexperienced practitioner, BOTOX® can actually give you wrinkles, the Daily Mail reports! Cosmetic experts have noted that knocking out some of the facial **muscles"** can bring others into play especially wrinkles across the top of the nose.

In a piece for the Journal of Cosmetic Dermatology, Dr David Becker, an assistant professor of dermatology at Weill Cornell Medical College in New York, observed that '**wrinkles** caused by untreated muscles of facial expression paradoxically can become **more prominent.** 'Paralysis of a set of muscles,' he suggests, 'might lead to recruitment of other muscle groups in an attempt to reproduce the conditioned activity being blocked - resulting in more prominent muscle activity in adjacent regions.'
http://www.marieclaire.co.uk/news/health/454268/can-botox-give-you-wrinkles.html

Other possible physical and physiological side effects include:

- **Lumps**
- **Blepharoptosis** (drooping of the upper eyelid)
- **Death - BOTOX® injections can kill you**
  http://news.softpedia.com/news/BOTOX®-Injections-Can-Kill-You-78531.shtml
- **Addiction**
  Doctors in the USA and the UK have reported that some patients "binge" on BOTOX® to the point where their faces look frozen. They refer to the term "Wrinklerexia" - when some BOTOX® devotees become so obsessed with their wrinkle-free image that they start seeing lines where there are none and binge on BOTOX® to obtain a freeze-frame face.
- **Wrinklerexia**
  http://www.medicalnewstoday.com/articles/158647.php
  BOTOX® bingers' obsession with 'freeze-frame' faces is leading worrying new 'wrinklerexia' trend
  The Harley Medical Group, which is the UK's largest cosmetic surgery provider, says that its surgeons are trying to curb the use of the anti-wrinkle product by recommending smaller doses of BOTOX® and has even turned away patients who demanded injections they don't need.
  /www.dailymail.co.uk/femail/article-1078067/BOTOX®-bingers-obsession-freeze-frame-faces-leading-worrying-new-wrinklerexia-trend.html

I have concluded that there are too many BAD references on BOTOX® to mention but here are a couple:

The Negative Side Effects of BOTOX®
http://www.livestrong.com/article/93774-negative-side-effects-BOTOX®-injections/
Allergen now battling 500 Lawsuits
http://blogs.wsj.com/health/2010/05/12/allergan-now-batting-500-in-BOTOX®-lawsuits/

BOTOX® Lawsuit Awards Virginia Man $212 million
http://breakinglawsuitnews.com/BOTOX® -lawsuit-awards-virginia-man-212-million/
Simon Cowell Left Disfigured by BOTOX® Treatment!
http://gossip.whyfame.com/simon-cowell-left-disfigured-by-BOTOX® -treatment-11538
Home BOTOX® Horror
http://www.sunnewsnetwork.ca/video/1176264539001
Bonnie Says: Don't Be A Victim Of Bad BOTOX® Like Megan Fox And Kate Gosselin!
http://www.hollywoodlife.com/2010/06/22/bonnie-says-dont-be-a-victim-of-bad-BOTOX® -like-megan-fox-and-kate-gossel/
Bad BOTOX® Failures
http://www.youtube.com/watch?v=UIZWBQ2J_Uc

My opinion of BOTOX®

I cannot dispute that it works to stop showing dynamic wrinkles in the short term but at what cost, especially in the long-term? It has only been around for 10 years. We were once told that BOTOX® was safe, but now we know **BOTOX® carries a Black Box Warning.** We were once told that it couldn't hurt you but now we know **BOTOX® can kill you.** We were once told that it could not migrate to the brain, but now we know **BOTOX® can migrate to the brain.** We were told that it wasn't addictive, BUT now we know **BOTOX® is addictive;** there is even a NEW medical term for it **"Wrinklerexia!"**

Facial expression is an essential part of communication; we are losing this innate ability with computer communication extending into our social lives; so perhaps in the end, it does not matter? Obviously, it begs the question then why would you bother with BOTOX®? If, at the end of the day, no one will see you, except those, (who -hopefully) love you beyond simple aesthetics?

Surely preventing wrinkles from forming in the first place is the answer? I am 56 and do not have a pronounced static wrinkle on my forehead or a frown line between my eyes because my facial muscles are all strong. ***Fitface is the answer.***

Tissue fillers

Various injectable products (I found a list of 140) that can be used to plump out the nose to mouth folds/ lines and deeper static wrinkles, or to enhance the lips for a plumper more youthful appearance.

The material for these fillers is derived from various sources - animal sources, donated human sources (yours or someone else's), or are they can be completely synthetic. Some of these cosmetic fillers are injected, while some are surgically implanted. The range in cost for one treatment can vary between a few hundred to a few thousand dollars.
http://www.plasticsurgeryinfo.com/cosmetic-fillers.shtml

Hyaluronic acid based fillers replenish lost volume such as Restylane, Perlane, Hydrafil and Juvederm. Some hyaluronic acid has been extracted from rooster combs. This injectable filler can be found in products like Restylane® and Captique®, both of which have received FDA approval.

Some points of interest are:
- Used cosmetically, there is a chance of an allergic reaction causing prolonged redness
- Most medical collagen is derived from young beef cattle (bovine) from certified BSE (bovine spongiform encephalopathy) free animals. Most manufacturers use donor animals from either "closed herds," or from countries, which have never had a reported case of BSE such as Australia, Brazil and New Zealand
- Porcine (pig) tissue is also widely used for producing collagen sheet for a variety of surgical purposes
- Alternatives using the patient's own fat, hyaluronic acid orpolyacrylamide gels, which are readily available
- Recently, human-derived injections like Plasmagel® and CosmoDerm® has joined the market
http://en.wikipedia.org/wiki/Collagen

Most of these cosmetic fillers can be classified as temporary (lasting a few weeks or months), semi-permanent (6-12 months) to permanent.

My opinion of fillers

Once again, I have to agree they work in the short term to puff up and push out the wrinkle or the fold. However, I repeat at what cost in the long run? Yes, fillers add volume, but this material has a certain weight, which over time the extra volume/weight "puff" stretches the skin beyond what nature intended. The stretch skin is permanently thinned. Thinner skin is less elastic. Therefore, in the long-term the filler makes the site of the injection more susceptible to aging as gravity will pull down the extra volume sooner than if it was left to nature! Ultimately; using fillers, results in dependency on fillers; this results in a self-defeating downward spiral. That is the reason celebrities' often look puffy, like chipmunks. Even Simon Cowell is looking cubby faced!

Full lips are the current fashion, and fillers have been used to plump out the lines above the lip and to make the lips fuller, such action often leads to a dependency on filler, to keep puffing out the lips because the stretch skin as become thinner and over time the person develops the "trout pout."

Duck Face Monsters
http://doodiepants.com/2012/03/03/collagen-lip-injections-duck-face-BOTOX® /

Fillers are often sold as a means of taking 10 years off the person, rolling back the clock to how they looked before, before they have aged ten years. Yes, one can look better in the short term, but "puffing out" a wrinkle is not nearly the same as ten years ago when there was not a line! It is convincing stuff when heard by a mature woman looking for a kind ear and the answer to aging. Sadly, once the cycle has begun, unless caught in the bud like most addictions; the seed is set, there follows a lifetime of fillers until cosmetic surgery is required as well the private sympathetic surgeon knows. In the meantime, he can and does expect future visits for treatment!

Fitface does prevent premature aging - prevention is always better than a cure.

Extremely invasive procedures
Surgical implants

These are generally small filler type implants to restructure the shape of the face. For example, a chin or cheeks implants. The operation to insert a chin implant is an otoplasty. The implant is made of synthetic material.

I can only say that I have met a woman in Palm Beach Florida, who clearly had cheek implants. Personally, I think she looked ridiculous, with high cheekbones when her face was never naturally supposed to be that shape! However, much worse, they didn't exactly move in tandem over her see through stretched skin. She looked pathetic, and I felt sad for her.

Cosmetic surgery

I don't think anyone takes on the pain, expense or risks of cosmetic surgery lightly. Although by the number performed perhaps I am wrong? But make no mistake, they are complex major operations.

Patients who seek consultation for facelift (rhytidectomy) are concerned about the aging of their facial features. The goal of the facial plastic surgeon is to determine the characteristics that are contributing to the patient's aging appearance and which of the characteristics are reversible. A comprehensive approach to the aging face may include endoscopic brow and/or midface lifting, eyelid modification surgery (blepharoplasty), chin and malar (cheekbone) implantation, and chemical/laser exfoliation in addition to rhytidectomy.

Understanding the patient's motivation for and expectations from the surgery is a key factor in successful surgery. Discussing such issues with the patient during the preoperative assessment is imperative.

The array of plastic surgery techniques used in face lifting surgery encompasses different depths of dissection and variation in approaches. These depths and approaches are denoted by terms such as: deep plane, subperiosteal, composite, various superficial musculoaponeurotic system SMAS (**sub-muscular aponeurotic system**) (imbrication or plication) procedures, approaches, subdermal, endoscopic, mini-incision, and laser assisted.

(SMAS is a layer of tissue that covers, surrounds and attaches to the deeper tissues and structures of the face and neck, including the entire cheek area).

Surgically elevating the SMAS layer helps to reposition all the tissues and structures of the face to a higher and more youthful point. This is usually accomplished using a technique called SMAS plication, (**folding** the SMAS back on itself).
http://plasticsurgery.about.com/od/glossary/g/smas.htm

Traditional facelift techniques, (such as SMAS imbrication or plication rhytidectomy) may adequately treat changes in the lower face caused by aging, such as jowling of the lower face or platysmal banding in the neck; however, these techniques do not adequately address aging changes due to ptosis (drooping or falling of the upper or lower eyelid) of midfacial structures and a deep melolabial fold.

The deep plane facelift was developed as a modification of standard facelift techniques to correct facial changes caused by aging that are due to ptosis of midface structures (malar fat pad). The deep plane facelift also attempts to correct deep nasolabial folds. Other techniques (excluding specific midface procedures) do not adequately address these problems.
http://emedicine.medscape.com/article/1294486-overview

Subperiosteal rhytidectomy can be used to reverse facial aging of the midfacial and lower facial region. The evolution of the facelift began with simple cutaneous remodelling and expanded to address subcutaneous layers. As techniques advanced, desire to improve the appearance of the nasolabial fold resulted in deep-plane rhytidectomy.
http://emedicine.medscape.com/article/841787-overview

My opinion on cosmetic facial surgery

Cosmetic surgery used to correct a deformity, a disfigurement, remove an unsightly mark, or change a really ugly facial feature or be used for reconstructive purposes following an accident or illness; it is and was marvellous. However, the whole industry has got out of hand. For me, I feel that to use the knife unnecessarily, purely for a minor imperfection or to try to reverse the natural aging is crazy. If you are a celebrity or a supermodel, then I suppose it is an acceptable requirement, but for the average person to put themselves through the whole ordeal just seems a complete waste of time, which I consider to be self-destructive or rather self-ham by proxy.

But, worse than being self-destructive; it is self-defeating - as to maintain the illusion of a more youthful appearance forever the whole process will need to be repeated within 7 to 10 years. The real crying shame is when you see a celebrity that has been known to have had a couple of facelifts they STILL look their age as soon as they give up the knife! Here I think instantly of Hilary Clinton, Tom Jones and Robert Redford, although I am sure, they had the best surgeon's money could buy. This is because with successive intervention the skin thins and becomes less elastic, which exacerbates aging. That's why; when the penny really drops they give up.

My only advice is if you are going to have a facelift, then please, please, please make sure you know what you are doing; be informed. Go to the best - you cannot afford a lifetime mistake or worse serious complications, nerve damage or death. Ask the right questions at the consultation and only deal directly with the surgeon not a sales girl at a clinic. Because if you don't know what you are doing and you are disappointed with the result, post cosmetic surgery (as apparently one in four are) you will have no one to blame but .yourself. Time and time again I read that the cosmetic surgeon blames the patient, citing that the client had too high expectations of what cosmetic surgery could do. So don't be a victim. Hear the truth, no what you had hoped or want to hear. They are not miracle workers. No surgeon can make a silk purse out of a sow's ear!

If you want to put yourself off for life (as I would hope you should) please just go to the internet and look at this link – or others, there are plenty to choose from!

50 Greatest Plastic Surgery Shockers
http://www.channel4.com/programmes/50-greatest-plastic-surgery-shockers/episode-guide/series-1/episode-1

The psychological effects of cosmetic surgery

There are negative consequences, and some people do become addicted to surgery and or BOTOX® injections. There have been many famous celebrities who have suffered this fate.

Negative Psychological Effects of Cosmetic Surgery
http://www.ehow.com/facts_4855098_negative-psychological-effects-cosmetic-surgery.html

The future for the cosmetics industry

I am glad that women and the cosmetics industry are addressing the real issue of healthy looking skin and the fundamental fact that skin grows from the inside out and needs to be nourished internally with nutrients delivered by the blood.

Finally, the beauty industry has woken up to the fact that women are becoming increasingly aware that "you are what you eat." That what you put in your mouth shows on your face (and body). To look good and glow, they now report that it is essential that you eat correctly. The future is not going to be about what you put on your skin to "look good" (so yesterday), but it will concentrate on the message that "It's what you put in your body that counts."

The cosmetics industry has joined forces with dieticians to bring to the table a whole host of new edible cosmetics. We have been aware for ages that vitamin supplements work (up to a point, some merely are never broken down and (therefore not ingested), rejected and instead expelled – flushed away) but the new idea is to put "beauty ingredients" such as aloe or collagen in drinks. Furthermore, to align branding of such newly generated products with spas or beauty salons to promote the extra health benefits such as oxygenated water.

The hype is good, but I don't agree. Sorry but for me, it's yet another gimmick. The body won't know what to do with the novel ingredients or how to break them down, let alone how to absorb them. So long as you eat a balanced diet, proteins, carbohydrates and fats that contain vitamins and minerals, with roughage then you can't go far wrong. If you start listening to your body and eat what it tells you to, rather than rely on recipes and diets (which we all know make us fatter), then you can't go far wrong.
http://www.brianmac.co.uk/nutrit.htm
http://www.mckinley.illinois.edu/handouts/macronutrients.htm

There are whole arrays of products in development from collagen marshmallows to sweets with extra estrogens that allegedly enhance your breast size! Some are even currently available in Japan.

The future is upon us

Women have long ingested vitamins pills to grown stronger nails, healthier hair and glowing skin. The next generation is all about edible cosmetics. I have found many articles which may increase your awareness and interest in nutricosmetics skingestibles, neutriceuticals and nutraceuticals and sippables.

Antioxidant-rich foods help to keep your skin healthy, but now these ingredients are offered in the form of supplements that aim to smooth wrinkles and leave your skin glowing. Sometimes called skingestibles or nutricosmetics, these pills, powders and ingestible potions contain a range of marine and plant compounds intended to improve skin's structure, appearance and tone.
ht/www.besthealthmag.ca/look-great/skin/could-a-pill-improve-your-skin

Edible cosmetics redefine inner beauty
Eat your way to clearer skin, healthier hair, and brighter eyes.
By Charlotte Andersen.
Beauty lotions and potions are so 2011. The newest way to make your skin glow, clear up acne, and brighten your eyes isn't with a little bottle of face cream but rather chocolate crème—as in the case of Borba's slimming chews and Frutel's new acne fighter both made out of, yes, chocolate. Apparently eating it, doesn't make you break out or gain weight! That is, if you buy into it?

Tanya Zuckerbrot, the official dietician of the Miss America pageant and co-creator of the edible Beauty Booster, says succinctly, "Juices have a ton of calories. Who wants to sacrifice their behind for their face?" Did we mention the Beauty Booster is calorie-and sugar-free?
http://www.shape.com/lifestyle/beauty-style/edible-cosmetics-redefine-inner-beauty

Proving beauty comes from within; the cosmetic industry joins the functional food market which has long been dosing food with vitamins, minerals and super foods for added nutrition-dense value, probiotic benefits, and wellness.
http://en.wikipedia.org/wiki/Probiotic

Beauty is skin deep

Now, "nutricosmetics" are applying the same principle to skincare. Beauty firms are including acai, goji berries, seathorn, green tea, seaweed, algae and other natural ingredients to edible products to enhance skin. So the idea is eat or drink for your health - everything from anti-aging to acne for a healthy complexion. My principals precisely!

While the jury is still out on whether they all work, several edible products claim of beautifying benefits, from snacks to beverages.
- Balance Bar's Nimble nutrition bar is formulated for the skin
- Deo Perfume Candy reportedly brings out a rosy fragrance through your pores
- Imedeen Tan Optimizer capsules claims to prevent sunburn
- Frutels **Chocolates** eliminate acne in a candy
- Votre Vu's Snap Dragon drinks beautify skin and health
- Herbasway's Beauty drinks for weight-loss and anti-aging
- Borba's Skin Balance waters available at Walgreens comes in four varieties to defy age, firm, clarify or replenish skin

Fashion designer Norma Kamali sells "liquid gold" for $45 for 200 millilitres in her New York City boutique. Basically its olive oil -- and she's a big fan, applying in to her skin and even brushing teeth with olive oil and cinnamon, which can eliminate bacteria.
http://www.treehugger.com/organic-beauty/edible-cosmetics-revolutionizing-beauty-product-industry.html

Home of the future Series 1 episode 5
http://www.channel4.com/programmes/home-of-the-future/4od
Back in 2003 an article was published in Beverage daily
'Skingestibles' blur the boundary
http://www.beveragedaily.com/Markets/Skingestibles-blur-the-boundary

The term nutricosmetics refers to nutritional supplements which can support the function and the structure of the skin. Many micronutrients have this effect. Vitamin C, for example, has a well established anti-oxidant effect that reduces the impact of free radicals in the skin. It also has a vital function in the production of collagen in the dermis. Other micronutrients e.g. some omega-3 fatty acids, carotenes and flavonoids protect the skin from the damaging effects of Ultraviolet (UV) light exposure, which may lead to accelerated skin aging and wrinkle formation. Natural oils such as Egg Oil (which contain Omega-3 and Omega-6 fatty acids), are often used topically as nutricosmetics.
http://en.wikipedia.org/wiki/Nutricosmetics

Nutraceuticals is a portmanteau of the words "nutrition" and "pharmaceutical" is a food or food product that reportedly provides health and medical benefits, including the prevention and treatment of disease. Health Canada defines the term as "a product isolated or purified from foods that is generally sold in medicinal forms not usually associated with food. A nutraceutical is demonstrated to have a physiological benefit or provide protection against chronic disease.
http://en.wikipedia.org/wiki/Nutraceutical

Fitface

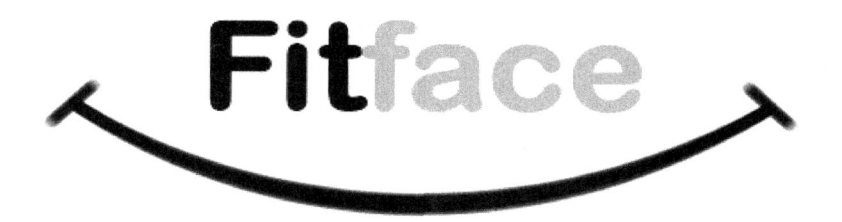

Fitface Facial Exercises

10 - minute face exercise routines

Part 2

Chapter 5

The exercises

Fitface guidelines
Your perfect face
Exercise programs
The weekly exercise routines
Daily routines
Skin care

How to do the exercises with photographs

If you have not already seen where your face muscles are take a look on one or both of these sites

Muscles of Facial Expression
Anatomy Tutorial
http://www.youtube.com/watch?v=Xmz3oLrnzBw

Artnatomy
Anatomical basis of facial expression learning tool
http://www.artnatomia.net/uk/index.html

The Fitface Toning Guidelines
Fitface puts health before beauty

Do not perform Fitface face or neck exercises if you have ever had any facial surgery, have used any BOTOX®, derma fillers or injectables without first consulting a dermatologist or your cosmetic surgeon (as applicable). Fitface toning exercises are preventative measures to avoid or postpone indefinitely invasive procedures.

1. Do not perform **Fitface toning** exercises for at least 6 months if you have had a laser or chemical peel as your skin will be fragile. Consult with your dermatologist or plastic surgeon as to precisely how many weeks or months it will be until your skin is fully healed.

2. **Do not exercise** if you have sunburn, the skin will be tight and fragile. Wait until the natural oils and body's own hydration returns to your skin.

3. **Don't exercise** if you are on prescribed pain killers as these can mask any of the warning signs to stop exercising.

4. Stop exercising immediately if you feel any pain or twinges and consult with a doctor.

5. Stop exercising if your muscles start to quiver. It is a sign that you are doing too much. Relax, there is always tomorrow.

6. **Do not exercise** your facial muscles if you feel tired, emotionally upset or if you are hung-over because you won't enjoy it and subconsciously you will remember the facial exercise as a negative experience. You can change brain plasticity either negatively or positively. Let the brain record the pleasant experience and the visible positive changes that will show on your face.

7. Be especially cautious with the neck exercises, take it very gently and **totally avoid them** if you experience any discomfort, aches or back problems. Don't bring

your head too far back, if it says, "Tilt your head", that's what it means. It does not mean to thrust your head as far back as is humanly possible!

8. When beginning to learn the face exercises start by using a mirror to execute the exercises correctly .When you become proficient at each of the exercises you will no longer need to look in the mirror, except to ensure that you are continually doing them correctly.

Notes

Start slowly; to get used to each of the exercises. If you find one too difficult at first, leave it out and come back to it later. Your muscle tone will improve over time and therefore, as with any exercise routine you will be able to do more, eventually.

Remember:

- Frequency is more important than the length of time spent on Fitface toning.

- Less is more; do no more than half an hour of continuous Fitface toning exercises in any one day especially when you are learning.

- Exercising must be fun, as well as good for you. Don't beat yourself up about not doing enough! Instead praise yourself up for what you can do and do do.

- Begin gently, if you find either the number of repetitions or the length of the hold time too difficult at first, relax. Move on. Over time, you may gradually work up to the required holding time or number of repetitions. If not, it is not the end of the world, just enjoy your routine.

- Always relax your shoulders.

- Always remember to breathe.

- The exercises are designed to be mixed and matched. **Do not just concentrate on your problem area or only a**

few exercises. IT WON'T WORK and this is the biggest mistake most people make.

- Maintain a healthy well rounded programme. Just as you don't work exclusively on one muscle at the gym (you work on the whole body) work your whole face with Fitface toning. **Should you wish to vary or expand your routine, additional exercises can be found in the original Fitface book, Fitface – Hands Free Facial Toning or the supplementary book Fitface Foundations.**

- Eventually learn a **Fitface toning** routine by heart so that you can perform it anywhere, even watching television or in the bath tub!

- Remember this for later. If on the first day, or the second day, or whenever you try **Fitface toning** and your muscles become sore, **stop**. Do not over do it. Come back. Try again. Start over. It is only natural that when you move muscles that have not been used much before, that once stretched they will feel sore. Soon they will rebuild and become stronger, tighter than ever before.

Your perfect face

When you begin to practice face exercises you will notice how your facial muscles move. With time you will become more and more self aware and more able to perfect your perfect face.

We all have a perfect face. The one you would like to show when you have your photograph taken but sadly don't always achieve it. To perfect your perfect face look in the mirror and pull your perfect face and then tweak it a little. Make the slight adjustment you want to.

Examples of adjustments
- Turn up the corners of your mouth
- Pull up under the eye
- Pull out eyebrows to stop the frown lines
- Pull from the temples to pull up and out the nasolabial folds

All muscles learn and with practice your perfect face will be the face you show the world. Your brain will make new neurological pathways that grow stronger with practice – practice really does make perfect. You can practice this exercise anytime, (on the train, driving, waiting in a queue (line)) whenever and wherever you want to.

Exercise programs

WEEKLY ROUTINE

Practice 5 times a week for 10 minutes a day to achieve the best results.

However, please do understand that **during the learning stage** this will probably take you 30 minutes! **Do start slowly; your face will let you know, what you can, and cannot do.**

I recommend performing the routine 5 times a week and then rest for 2 days. The routine is flexible you can miss a day, a week, or even a month but I would never want you to stop completely, forever. If you go on holiday/vacation take a break but don't stop forever. However, you may find that once you get into the groove and have seen the results for yourself you will do it secretly) even on holiday! I remember my friends bulling me when I did – yet now they say, "I looked at you and you have no wrinkles on your forehead, why? – Guess!

Even if you do stop for ages because you are ill there is nothing better for you than to get back in shape, both mentally and physically. If you don't use it, you will lose it. Be it an old lady - who has had a fall but was active. She starts to sit in a chair all day (to recover slowly) and pretty soon she is too tired to walk outside; within six months she is too lazy to walk 100 yards, let alone 300 yards and less than a year later she can't walk inside a hospital and needs a wheelchair - and now expects to be pushed! "If you don't use it; you lose it", it really is that simple.

The bigger picture is that the problem begins far earlier. It is a slow process for the body to degenerate from the young lady who can't be bothered to exercise, to the fat old lady who can't be bothered to walk; to wearing nappies and death. But it takes about 85 years! The moral is to start young to stay young.

What has this got to do with facial exercise you might ask? Well much depends on how much you care about the way you look. Whether you want a life of nothingness for years or still have hopes, dreams, ambition and want to make the most of the life you have. If you want to do nothing then I doubt that you would have purchased this book in the first place! This book is aimed at people between 30 and 50 who don't want to give up on life, at least not just yet!!

The most important thing for your successful facial exercise habits, is to establish a routine - that you can live with and stick to it

It is up to the individual, to fit Fitface in, within their normal routine. Much depends on your individual life style and whether or not you wear makeup and if so, whether or not you are prepared to let others see you "messed up", say in the gym (I have not done facial exercises with makeup only in the photos)!

Make face exercise your time.

Just like making up or taking a shower, fit it in somehow but don't make it a pain, it's something good for you. Think of it as investing **now,** for your future happiness.

The day afterwards

I have always found that I look better the day after I do facial exercise. Possibly because I have done them for so long that I can see the tightness and do not want to break it down/relax the tone on the day/evening/night when I am going out for a special occasion. That day, I give facial exercise a miss. It sounds like I'm hooked (guess, I sort of am) but I and you, must understand that the body needs time to repair and heel to build strong muscles.

DAILY ROUTINE

The warm up consists of 2 minutes, the exercises are 5 to 6 minutes in duration and the cool down is 1-2 minute which makes between 9 and 11 minutes but it is not an exact science. I have included an extra minute for turning pages. But no matter however many times I practice this routine it is never takes exactly the same time, even though I use a clock! The only other equipment you will need is a mirror.

The daily routines

Keep it simple, as simple as- 1-2-3

1. Warm up
2. Exercises
3. Cool down.

Timing each exercise

Each exercise is about a minute, unless stated to the contrary. Many exercises are grouped in sets of threes this is so as to build up intensity in the shortest possible time.

Don't be too hard on yourself, relax about the specific timings. They are all meant to be a guide to be loosely adhered to after you are comfortable with the exercise and the routines.

To count a second:

I use the method of saying "One thousand and" before the number - to take up one second in time. To test yourself for your personal accuracy:

1. Find a clock with a second hand
2. Start counting when the second hand is on the hour
3. Count like this – say, "One thousand and one, one thousand and two, one thousand and three etc up until you reach 15
4. Check your time against the clock; hopefully it is approximately 15 seconds. If not adjust your timing as necessary.

The holds

Please, be sensible if it says 1 minute but you can only hold for 10 seconds just stop and start again as many times as necessary within the minute

The warm up

The first part lasts 2 minutes and comprises of 16 different exercises.
This section has been; specifically designed to be a whole face and neck warm-up to get the blood flowing in order to nourish the cells with oxygen and nutrients.

After the **warm-up** your face may itch. This is not a bad sign! It just means that your blood has reached/circulated to those areas that it doesn't normally do. If this bothers you, either just wriggle your face or relax your head and gently shake you face from side to side for a few seconds. Alternatively, at this point you may want to scream to stretch your face and neck muscles; all this is the face/body's normal reaction to having activated those sluggish, underused neck and facial muscles

The daily exercises

The next section or mid section - show the specific face exercises designed to concentrate on one part or area of the face. Please remember: that most of the facial muscles work in sync, therefore, work one and you work them all, or far more than is superficially obvious.

I have tried to make them a combination of isometric and isotonic eccentric exercises. but in the face, to be specific about any type of exercise is practically impossible. As a very loose, general (broad) term I have interpolated:

- **Isotonic concentric** – to be a flowing movement
- **Isotonic eccentric** – to be as the slow deceleration of a movement
- **Isometric** to be a static hold

The first day you practice you may feel like giving up and each exercise may take 10 times the length of time it is supposed to take but don't be discouraged. Even when you think you have the hang of each exercise after the first week it may still take you double or even triple the time permitted but do not worry, in no time at all it will become second nature to you. Be patient with yourself, it will come. It's like anything else, practice makes perfect - remember your first driving lesson!!!

The cool down

To relax those muscles that you have just worked to stimulate blood flow once again as people tend to hold their breath and slightly stress when exercising especially in the learning phases.

Post exercise

Just like after a body workout or any other form of exercise, the next day, your face may feel tight, strained or stretched. Don't overdo it, like all exercise listen to your body, but in this case your face.

THE" Hands Free" WARM UP
16 exercises
2 minutes

Isotonic concentric exercises designed to enable the facial muscles to go through their full range of motions to ensure the blood circulates from the forehead to the base of the neck

Perform each exercise 3 times

All 16 exercises are to be completed within 2 minutes

Note: Exercises 1 -10 seem to be faster, than 11-15

1. Eyebrow lifts – up n' out
2. Eyes – up and down
3. Eyes – side to side
4. Under eye lifts – up and down
5. Bunny noses – up and down

6. Nose tip – pull down
7. Nostril flares
8. Mouth circles – forwards
9. Mouth circles – backwards
10. Wide smiles – to widest
11. Say "Oh"
12. Stick tongue out
13. Neck – up and down
14. Face – side to side
15. Head circles – clockwise
16. Head circles – anticlockwise

Preferably start the warm up with a clean moisturised face; it will make you feel better. It's a little like changing into your workout clothes to do your body exercises, it puts you in the mood, even though many you could do in stocking feet wearing a dress.

THE EXERCISES
30 "hands free" exercises
6 minutes

The exercises mainly comprise of isometric static hold exercises to strengthen facial muscles combined with isotonic exercises and a few more difficult isotonic eccentric exercises.

I have very roughly divided the 30 exercises to represent 5 areas of the face, or one section for each of the five weekdays; (with 6 exercises in each section)

Either do **one face section a day** - consisting of 6 exercises (in rotation) or a **specific numbered exercise** each day. For example; perform all number 1's on Monday, all number 2's on Tuesday etc. Alternatively, choose to do **one face section a day**. Example: Whole face Monday, then Mouth (lower face) on Tuesday etc

For added variety; you may prefer to do alternative routines each week beginning with a face section a day (for the first week – of 5 days) followed by the numbered exercises for 6 days, etc.

However, you can mix and match at will. The possible combinations of 5 days with 6 exercises in each are 15,625 plus the 16 warm up and 2 cool down exercises! Therefore, for simplicity the book follows the following most effective pattern.

Most of the face muscles are interlinked in one way or another. For best results and the most intense workout concentrate on one area a day for each of the five days a week that you intend to exercise.

Please Note:

You will not be doing yourself any favours if you push yourself too much and try to perform the more strenuous pulls before you are ready.

Face exercise routines.

There are 5 sections, which are:

1. Whole face
2. Mouth Lower – (Chin, jaw line jowls)
3. Eyes
4. Mouth Upper –(Nasolabial folds/cheeks)
5. Neck

WHOLE FACE

1. Scream n stare
2. Scream n screw up face
3. Scream n under eyes up
4. Whole face lift
5. Whole face taut
6. Your perfect face

MOUTH (lower face)

1. Mouth corners - smile n hold
2. Mouth corners - smile n kiss
3. Mouth corners - smile n cheeks up
4. Chin – grin
5. Chin – hard grin
6. Chin – tongue press

EYES

1. Bags up
2. Ultra stares
3. Eye circles
4. Eyes - in and out
5. Winks
6. Eye pulls

MOUTH (upper face)

1. Nasolabial folds – tongue holds
2. Nasolabial folds – tongue sides in n out
3. Nasolabial folds – surprised snarls
4. Cheeks – smile
5. Cheeks – open smile to whistle
6. Cheeks – open smile n cheeks up

NECK

1. Sad face jowls
2. Nods
3. Back kisses
4. Side flops
5. Twist
6. Décolletage pull ups

THE COOL DOWN
4 "hands free" exercises
1 - 2 minutes

Select any two of the exercises below and divide your remaining time performing each one.

The following day select a different two

1. Ear rubs
2. Hair pulls
3. Head flops (between knees if seated)
4. head claws

GENERAL INFORMATION

Begin with a clean moisturised face if possible – (perspiration after a workout is okay). If you are wearing makeup the face exercise won't feel good and it will almost certainly mess up your makeup, so take it off. If you are in hurry just use a cleaning wipe followed by a moisturiser.

Always start with teeth and lips loosely closed together, unless otherwise stated.

Do not worry about the exercises, if you can't do one move or cut down the time. Its suppose to be fun, don't take it too seriously

10 minute routines

Learn how to do each of the warm up exercises. Then (instead of having to look at each book page) you can just check that you remember them all from the list overleaf entitled the
Two minutes "hands free" warm up exercises

After which: **Choose from either:**

Or
    Doing all of the 5 exercise for one section/part of the face

    Doing all of a specific number of the 6 exercises each day
    For example: On Monday do all exercises numbered one and on Tuesday do all exercises marked number two.

To end the daily practise, follow with two facial exercises from the selection of four cool **down** exercises.

SKIN CARE (My routine)
In the morning

Firstly, I wash, or rather I splash on tepid tap water. I may sometimes do my eye corners with a cotton bud dipped in the tap water

Next, I use a product that I invented. It is a spray concoction - I have a small spray plastic bottle filled with tap water, to which I have added a couple of drops of my very basic (dermatological, perfume free – hypoallergenic, E45) moisturising lotion which I have shaken up (to dissolve). However, without preservatives it can go off and start to stink, at that point I obviously start a fresh with a new bottle.

I make a fresh batch weekly.

I have tried a 'bought' rose water spray that smells much nicer than my concoction but I am not sure that it works just as well. But, I've run out and can't readily find it locally so my concoction works fine.. Recently I found a new moisture boost hydro mist by Simple an English brand

I have found that mountain spring water aerosol spray water is no good despite what it says on the can. As it is 100% pure water and as it evaporates off of the skin it takes with it your natural essential skin lipids. If you do use a water spray it is fine, just so long as you then apply a layer of your moisturiser to trap the water in your skin but do not use the spray alone.

Note: Even after my skin care routine I use this spray often as a means of hydration, for example on an aeroplane, even over makeup

After the spray, I then apply a thin, top coat of E45 moisturise and that's that. I am ready for the world, or to then apply makeup.

At night

Let your skin breathe as much as possible.

I am **not** a fan of night creams. I don't use one. They are too heavy and block the body's natural way of expelling perspiration and toxins. I use nothing, not even a moisturiser!

However, my routine is unrealistic for most women (or certainly was for me when I was in the corporate world). Therefore, I would suggest that you remove your makeup at night with either a gentle lubricant or wipes and then TRY to put on just a dash of light moisturiser on top. That way when you wake up in the morning, you will not have to "scrub" and stretch your skin (beyond an inch of its natural life) with hundreds of lotions and potions.

Perfect skincare is more difficult, especially as you age.

Once a week I will gently exfoliate where necessary with E45 (or any light moisturising cream). I place a small amount of that moisturising lotion on a cut off piece of a cheap (Poundland/The dollar store) exfoliating glove/mitt. Or occasionally I use an exfoliation wipe but unfortunately the good ones that are cheap and super gentle are very hard, almost impossible, to find.

I wish I could do nothing at all because the skin will look after itself better than I can. In the past, I have discovered that when I'm on some sort of an adventure in some foreign land unable to do anything to my skin for an extended period of time (such as a month) my skin is unbelievably naturally radiant. AMAZING! My skin looks perfect. This is also borne out by my mother of 82 who DOES NOTHING (and I mean NOTHING – despite my saying how disgusting it is)! She does not even wash with water but has PERFECT SKIN. She will do her eyes (as I do) with a cotton bud but she, unlike me, uses boiled, cool water. She rests her case! We endlessly discuss her skin but I, or rather my face, has become SO accustomed to a mild moisturiser that I feel naked without it. She does admit that it was not until she was about 60 that she gave up on her past favourites' of Anne French Cleansing Milk and Oil of Olay.

Photographs

All photographs were taken by me, Charlotte Hamilton, the author on my personal camera at home in my bedroom. Hence they are completely natural, with highlighter to show you that dynamic winkles do form when you exercise your face. But because exercise works all the muscles and builds collagen potential dynamic wrinkles do not become static wrinkles. A strong toned face prevents wrinkles.

Two minutes "hands free" warm up exercises

Eyebrow lifts – up n' out

Eyes – up and down

Eyes – side to side

Under eye lifts - up and down

Bunny noses – up and down

Nose tip – pull down

Nostril flares

Mouth circles – forwards

Mouth circles – backwards

Wide smiles – to widest

Say "Oh"

Stick tongue out

Neck – up and down

Face – side to side

Head circles – clockwise

Head circles – anticlockwise

Warm Up
1
Eyebrow lifts - up n' out

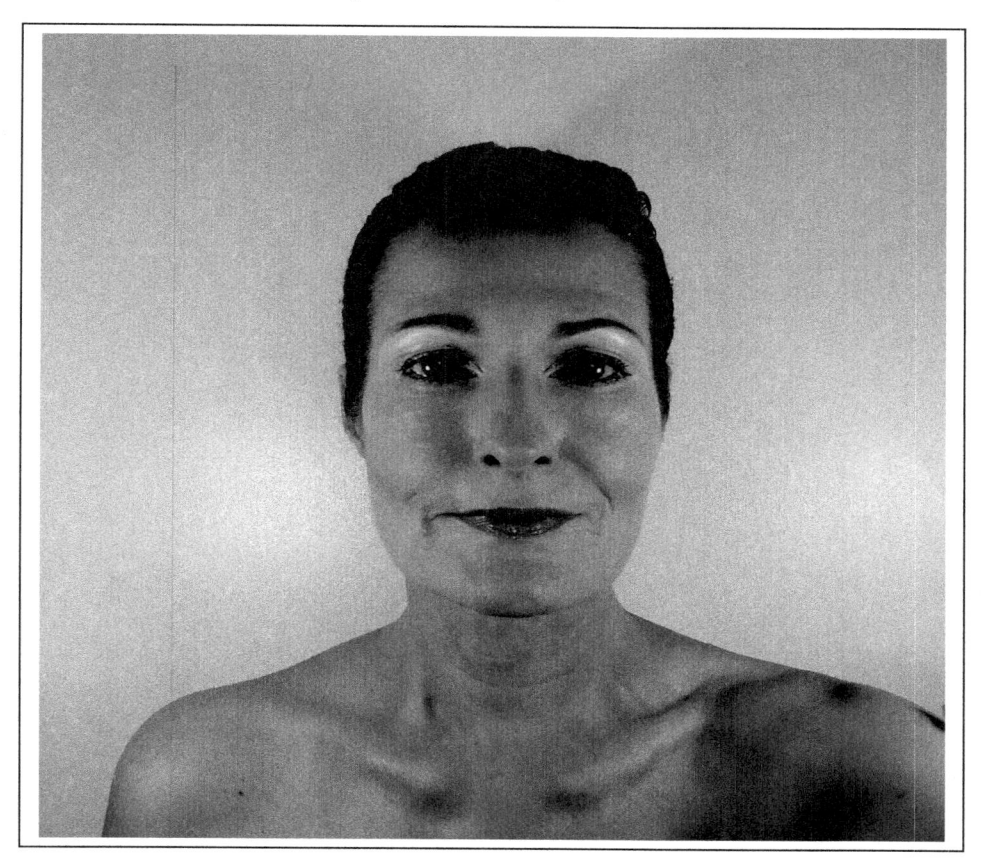

Move your eyebrows up as high as possible and pull them out and then
Relax

Repeat 3 times

Warm Up
2
Eyes -- up and down

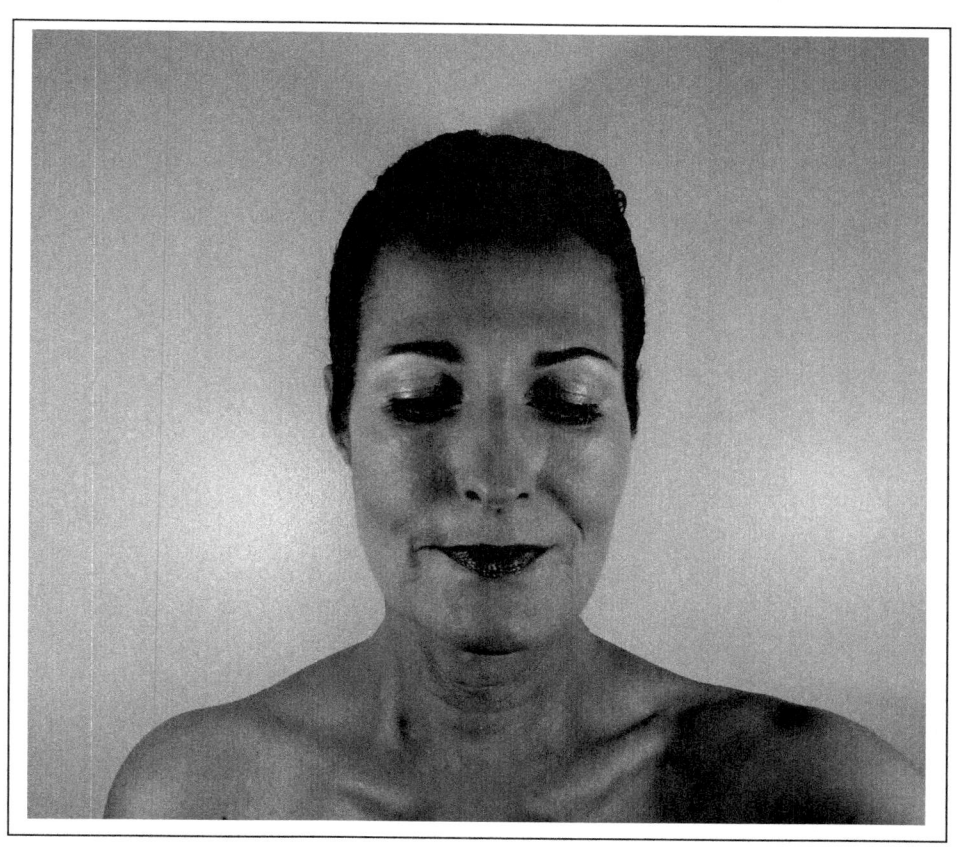

Look up as high as possible lifting your eyebrows up then
Look down as low as possible, looking to the outside corners

Repeat 3 times

Warm Up
3
Eyes – side to side

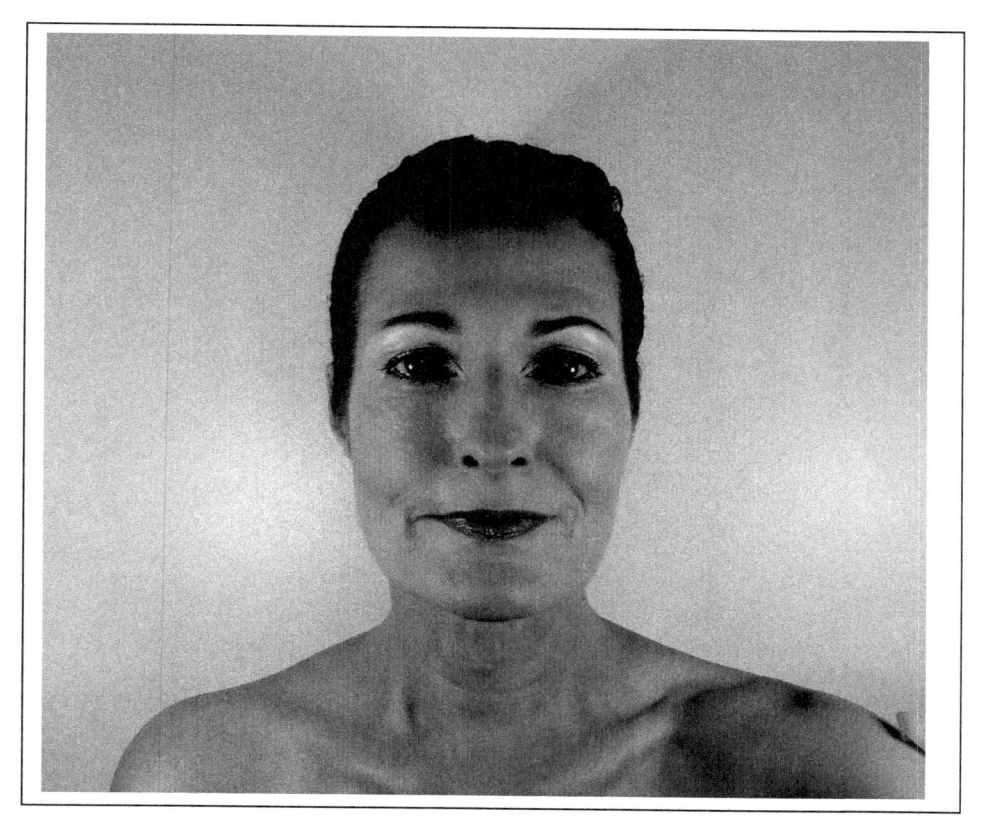

Look left as far as possible then draw your eyes over to look right as far as possible

Repeat 3 times

Warm Up
4
Under eye lifts – up and down

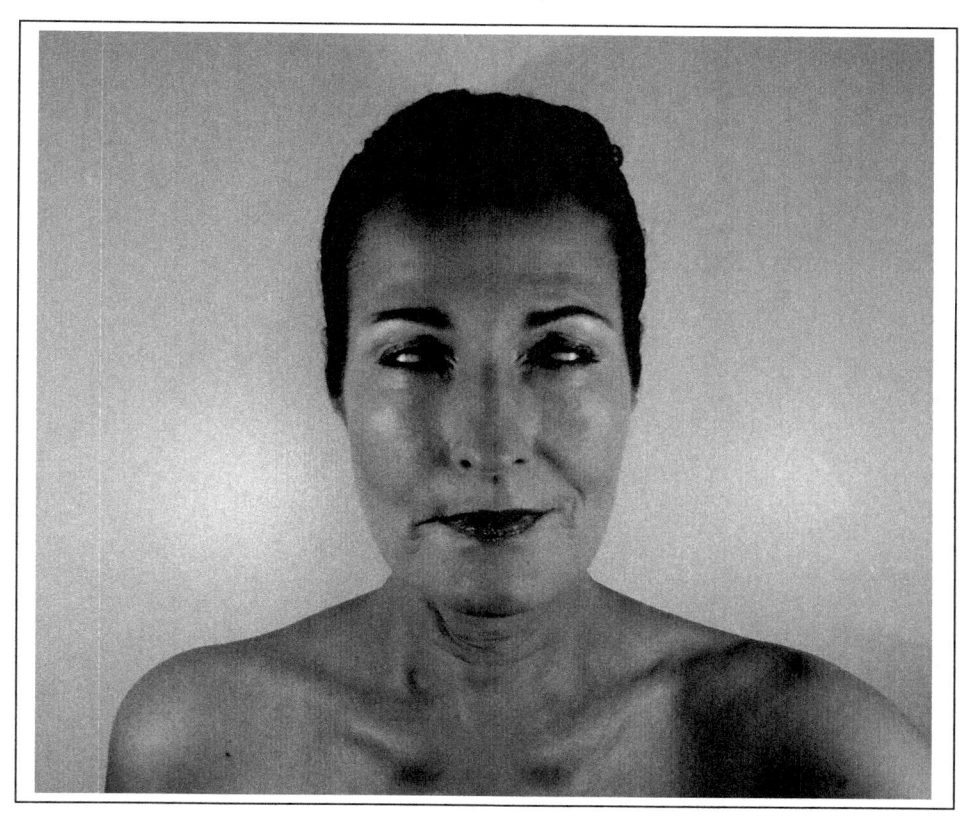

Pull up your under eyelids to close your eyes pause and then Release

Repeat 3 times

Warm Up
5
Bunny noses – up and down

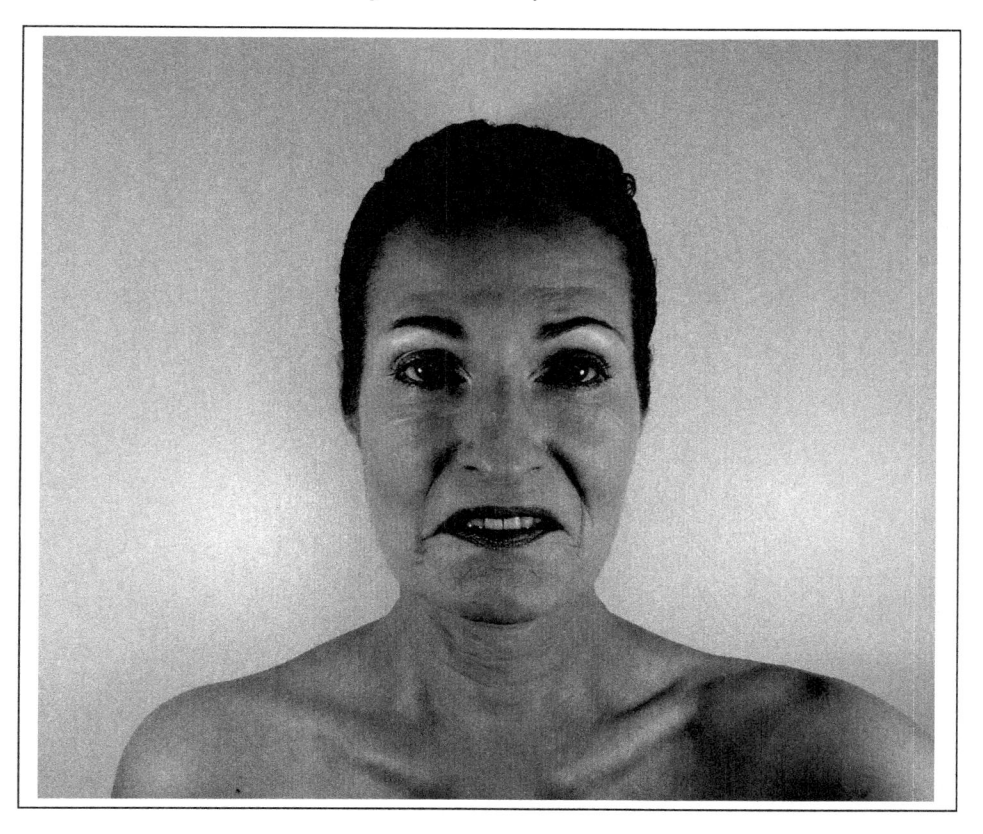

Start with teeth together
Raise the sides of your nose as high as possible, pause and then drop them

Repeat 3 times

Warm Up
6
Nose tip – pull down release

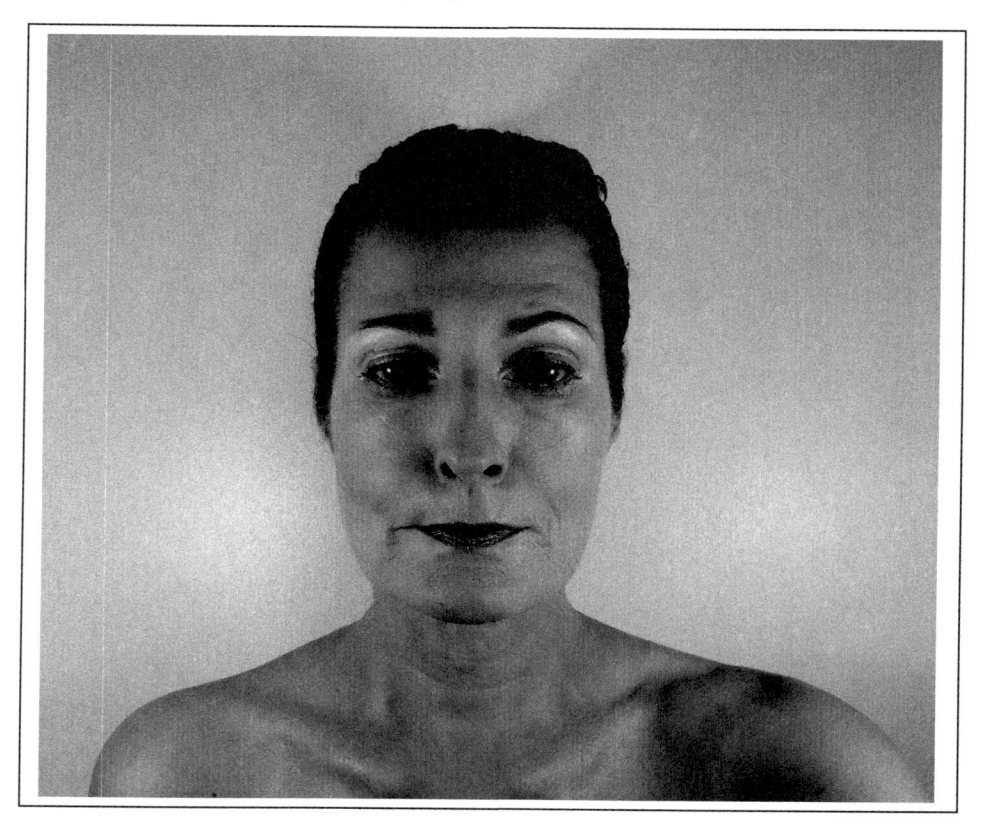

Pull down your nose as far as possible, and then release

Repeat 3 times

Note:
Hold your eyebrows level.

Warm Up
7
Nostril flares

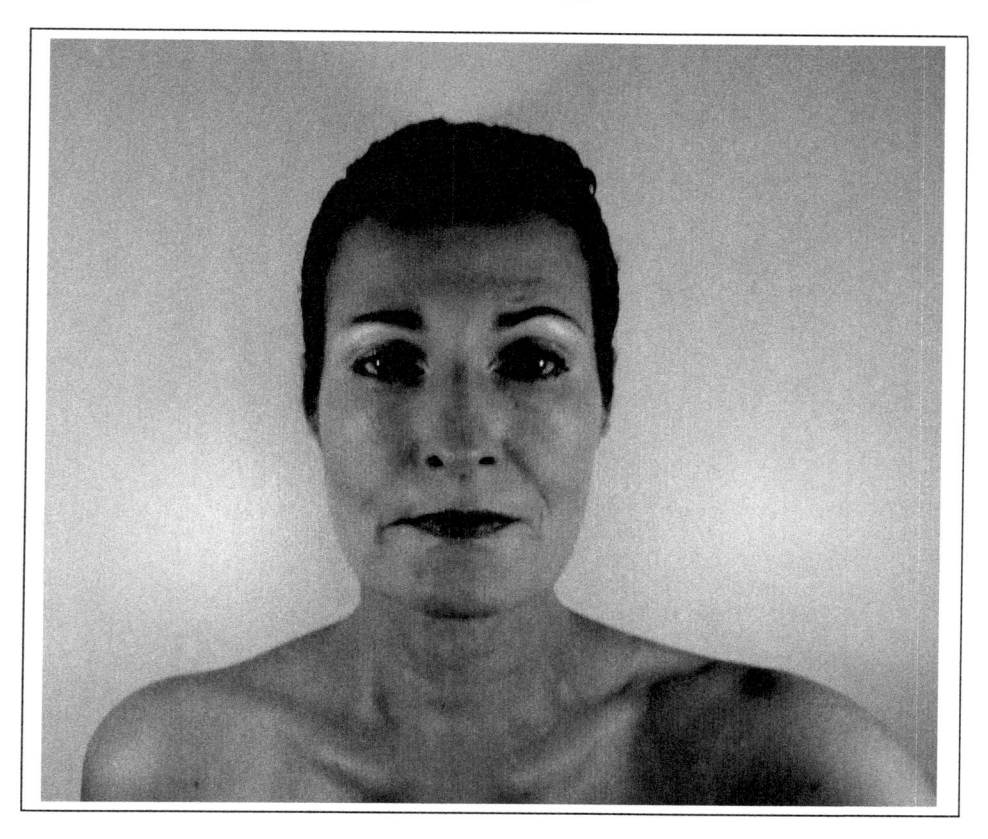

Flare the sides of your nose out, hold for a second then release

Repeat 3 times

Note:
If you find it difficult, blow through your nostrils

Warm Up
8
Mouth circles - forwards

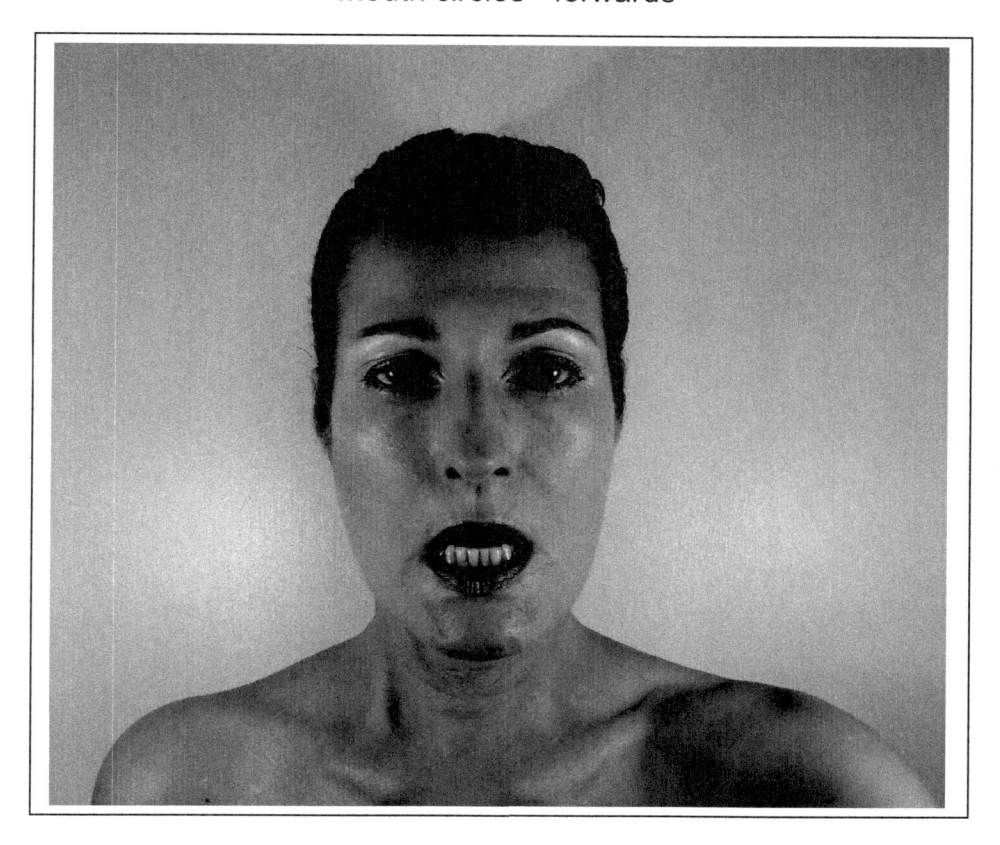

Open your mouth and then move your jaw forwards naturally in a wide open circular motion

Repeat 3 times

Note:
Your mouth should be shaped like a circle, an "O"

Warm Up
9
Mouth circles – backwards

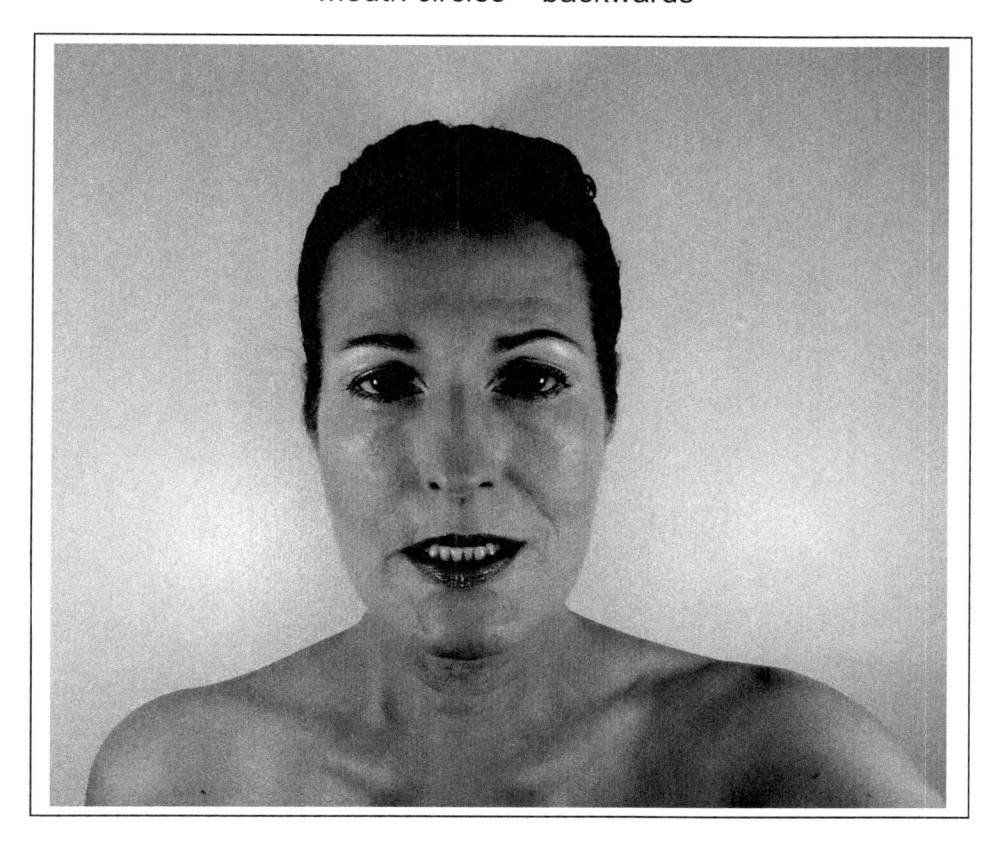

Open your mouth and then move your jaw backwards naturally in a wide open circular motion

Repeat 3 times continuously

Note:
Your mouth should be shaped like a circle, an "O"

Warm Up
10
Wide smiles – to widest

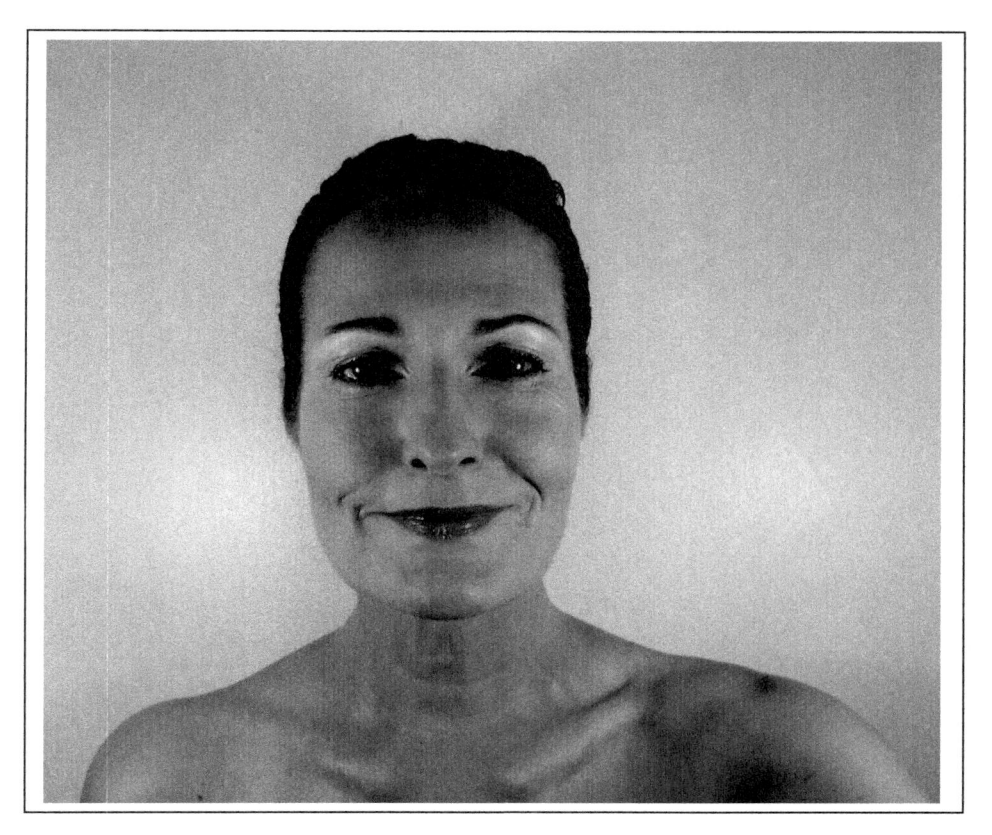

Teeth and lips together
Smile as wide as possible pulling up the corners of the mouth to the eye corners, pause then
Relax

Repeat 3 times

Warm Up
11
Say "Oh"

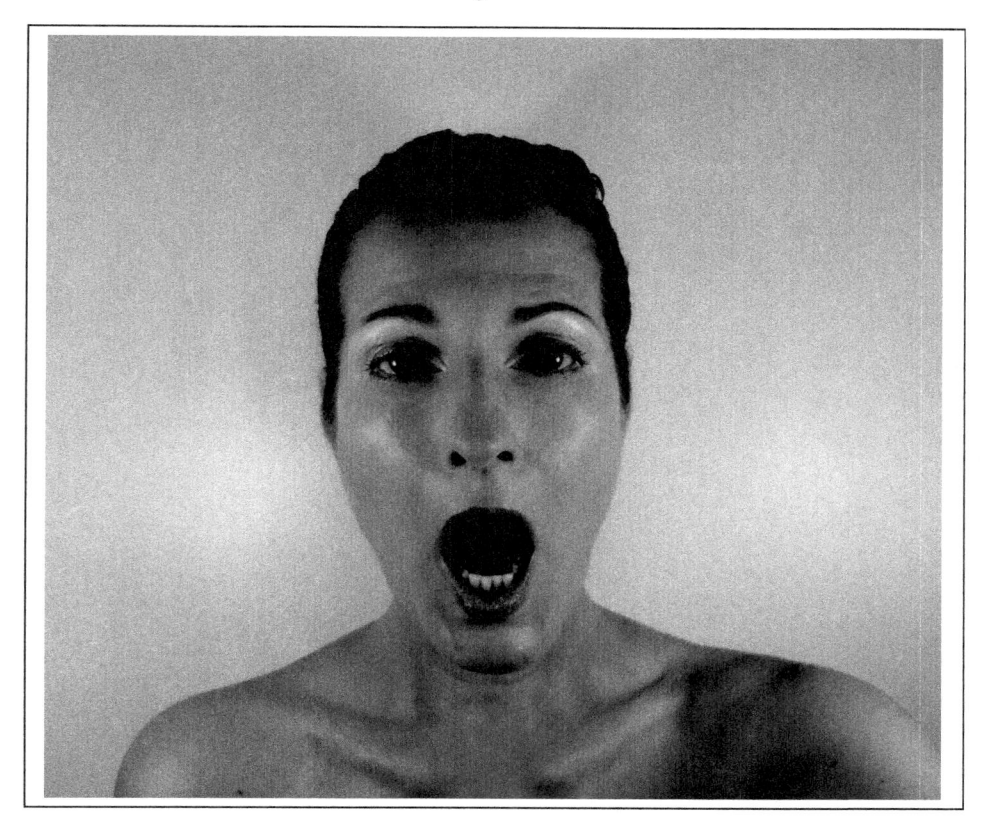

Open your mouth as wide as possible and say "Oh", pause, hold taut and then release

Repeat 3 times

Note:
You can just say "Oh" to yourself! Your mouth shouldl be an oval shape.

Warm Up
12
Stick tongue out

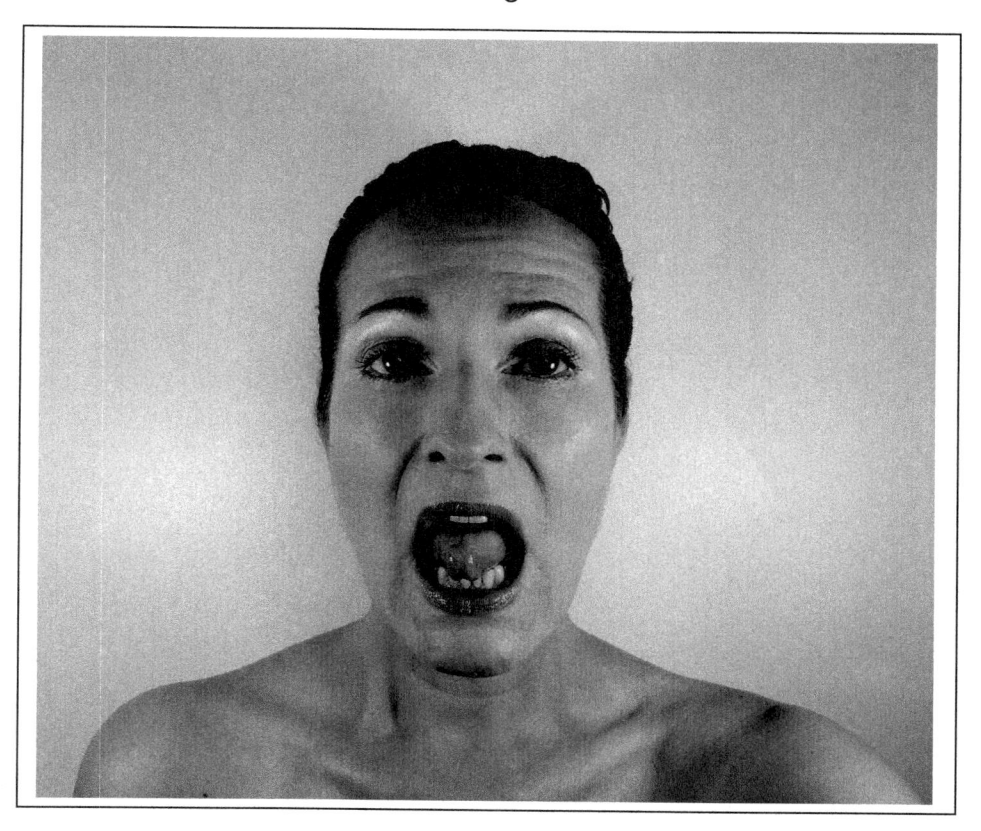

Stick your tongue out as far as possible, eyebrows high and pause and then
Relax

Repeat 3 times

Note:
Your neck muscles should stand out
The sides of your mouth should feel pulled.

Warm Up
13
Neck – up and down

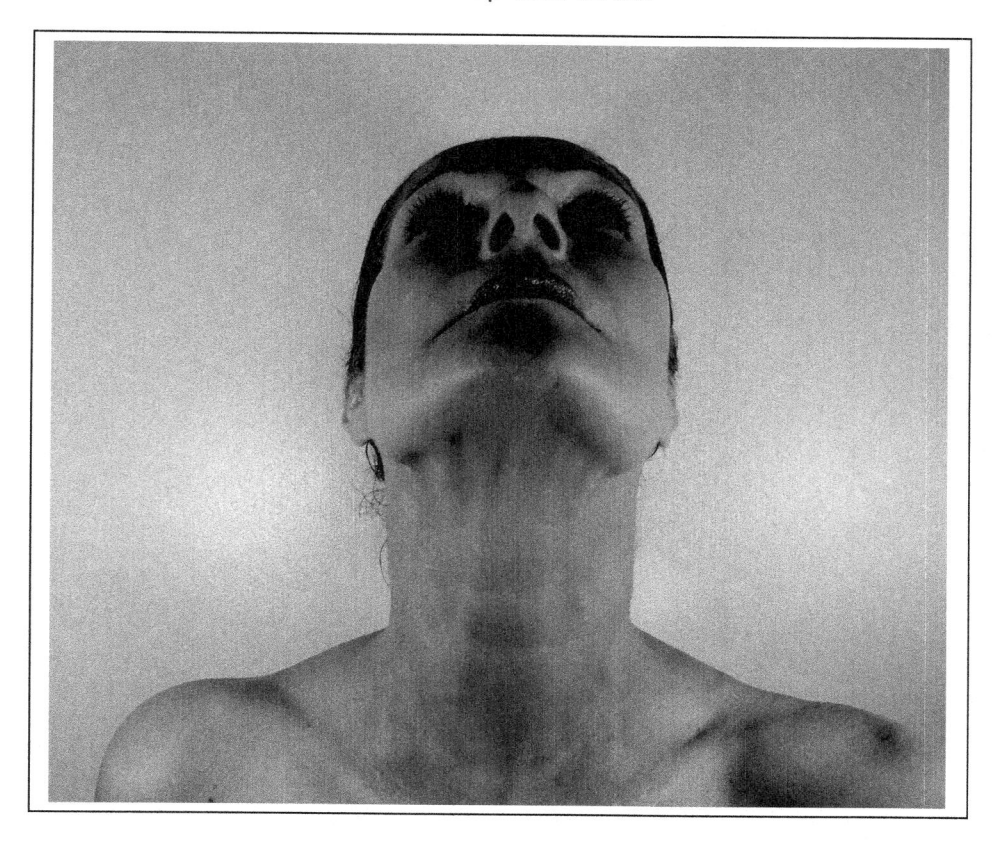

With your head in a central, natural position, teeth and lips together in a straight smile and relaxed shoulders
Gently and slowly drop your head backwards and look up at the ceiling, next
Gently bring your head slowly forward and extend so that your chin touches your décolletage/chest then
Gently raise your head back up to a level position

Repeat 3 times

Note:
Omit any and all neck exercises if you feel any abnormal (to you) twinges.

Warm Up
14
Face side to side

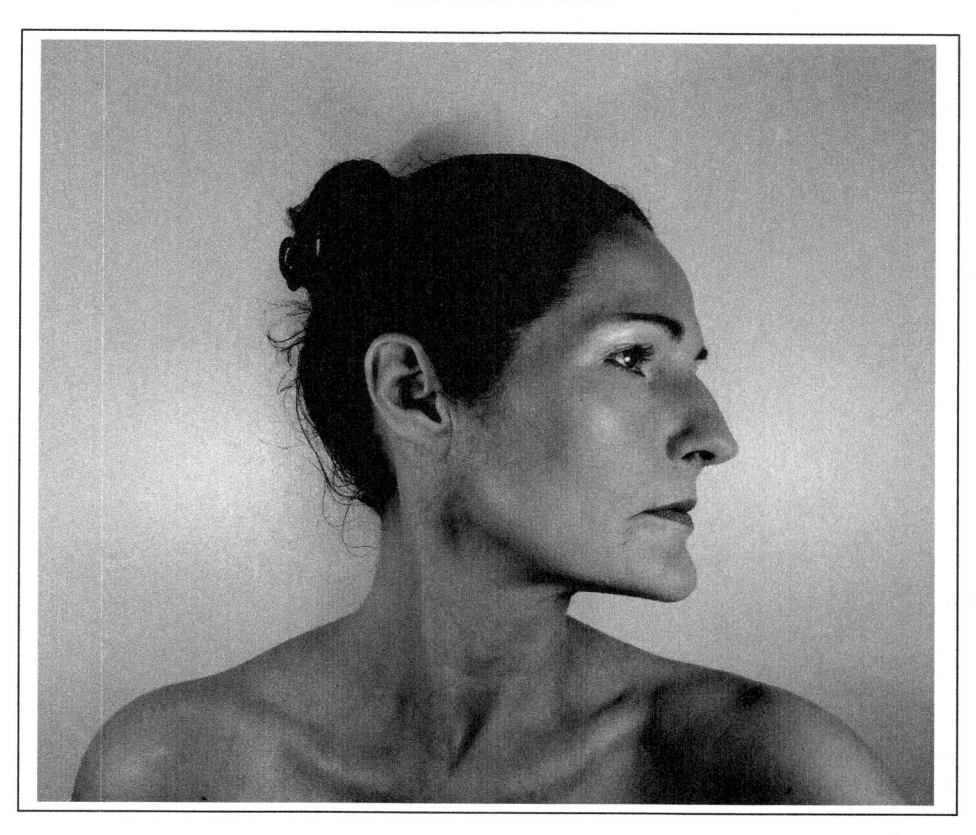

With your head in a central, natural position, teeth and lips together in a straight smile and relaxed shoulders

Turn your head slowly to look left as far as possible then
Bring your head back to the centre next
Turn your head slowly to look as far right as possible, return to centre

Repeat 3 times

Note:
This should be a fluid, continuous movement
Keep your shoulders down.

Warm Up
15
Head circles – clockwise

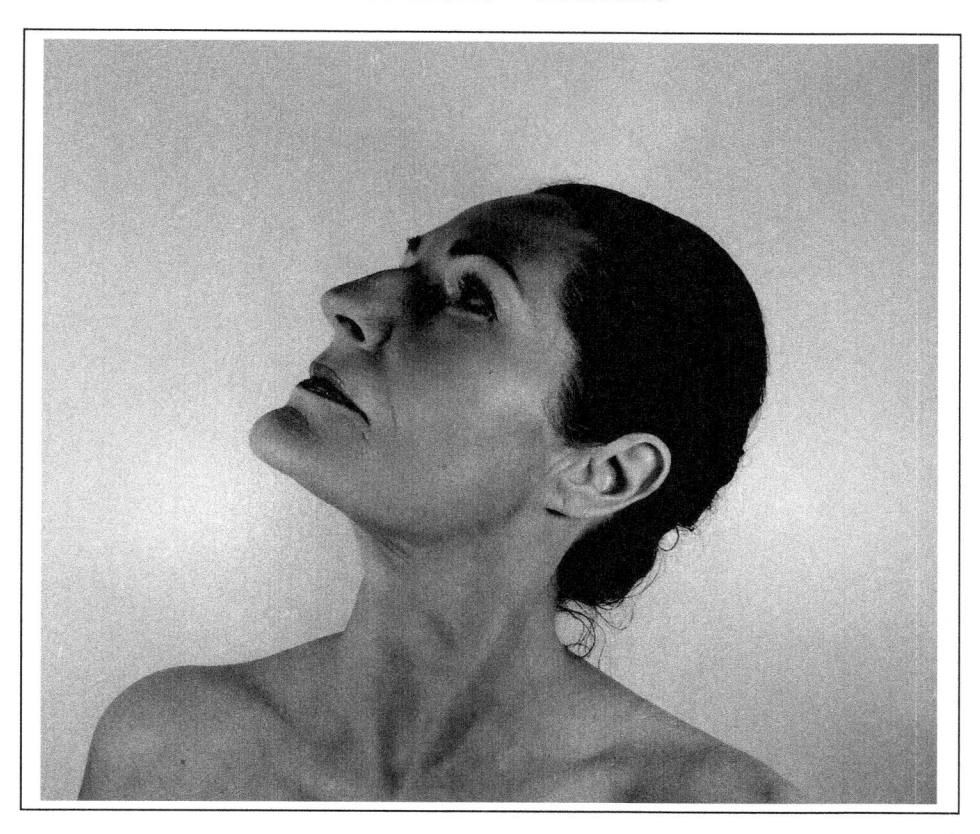

Looking forward, (relax your shoulders) with your head in a central, natural position, teeth and lips together in a straight smile.

Naturally drop head, gently circle up to the left, flow up to the top and gently drop your head to the right, and then slowly release down to the chest

Repeat 3 times

Note:
This should be a fluid, continuous movement.

Warm Up
16
Head circles - anticlockwise

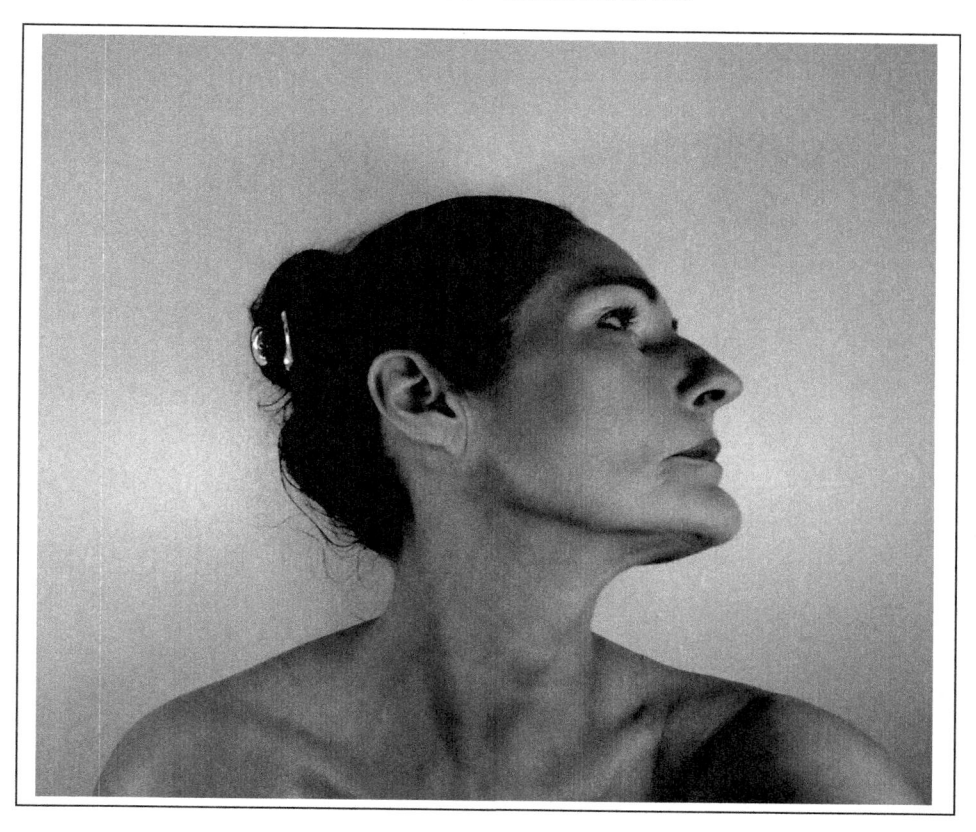

Looking forward, (relax shoulders) with your head in a central, natural position, teeth and lips together in a straight smile.

Naturally drop head, gently, circle up to the right, and flow up to the top and gently drop your head to the left and then slowly release down to the chest

Repeat 3 times

Note:
This should be a fluid, continuous movement.

Exercises
WHOLE FACE 1
Scream n stare

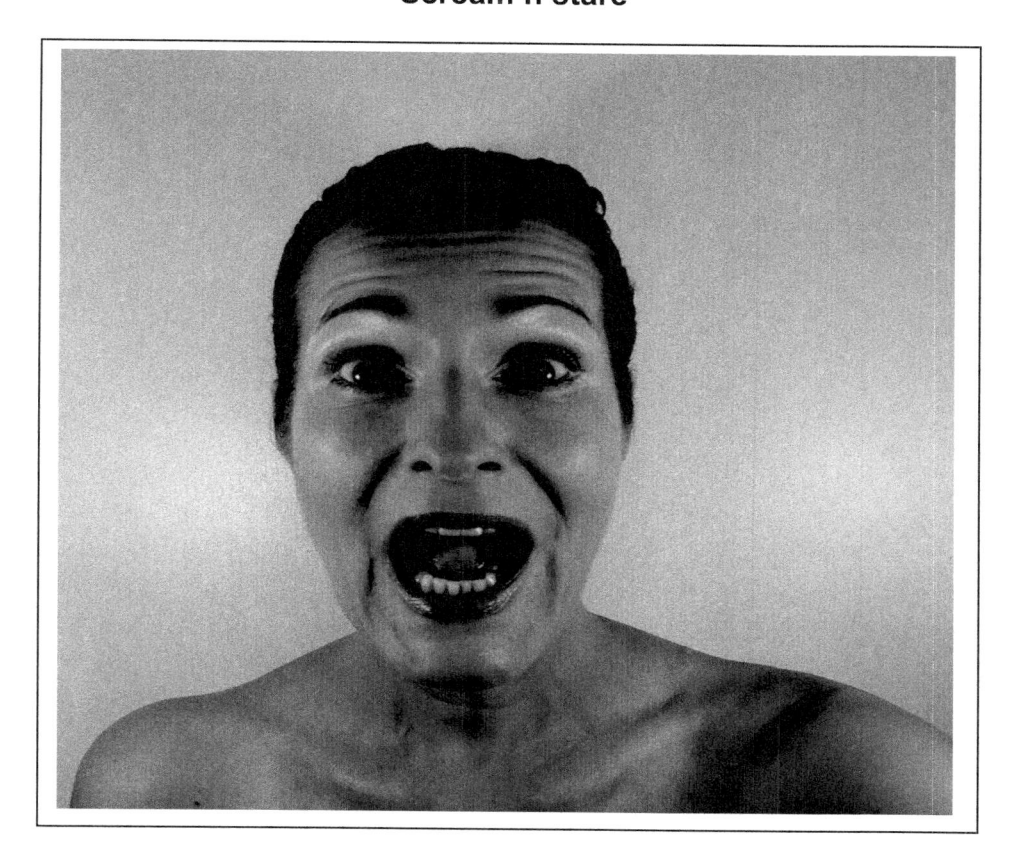

Scream with a big wide open mouth shaped like an "O" and raising your eyebrows high, opening out every muscle in your face pause, then
Stare
Pull every facial muscle back and hold taut

Hold: 1 minute

Note:
Your will feel your eyes bulging forwards in the stare but you will not be able to hold the stare for a minute so blink when necessary and stare again but hold the scream taut.

Exercises
WHOLE FACE 2
Scream n screw up face

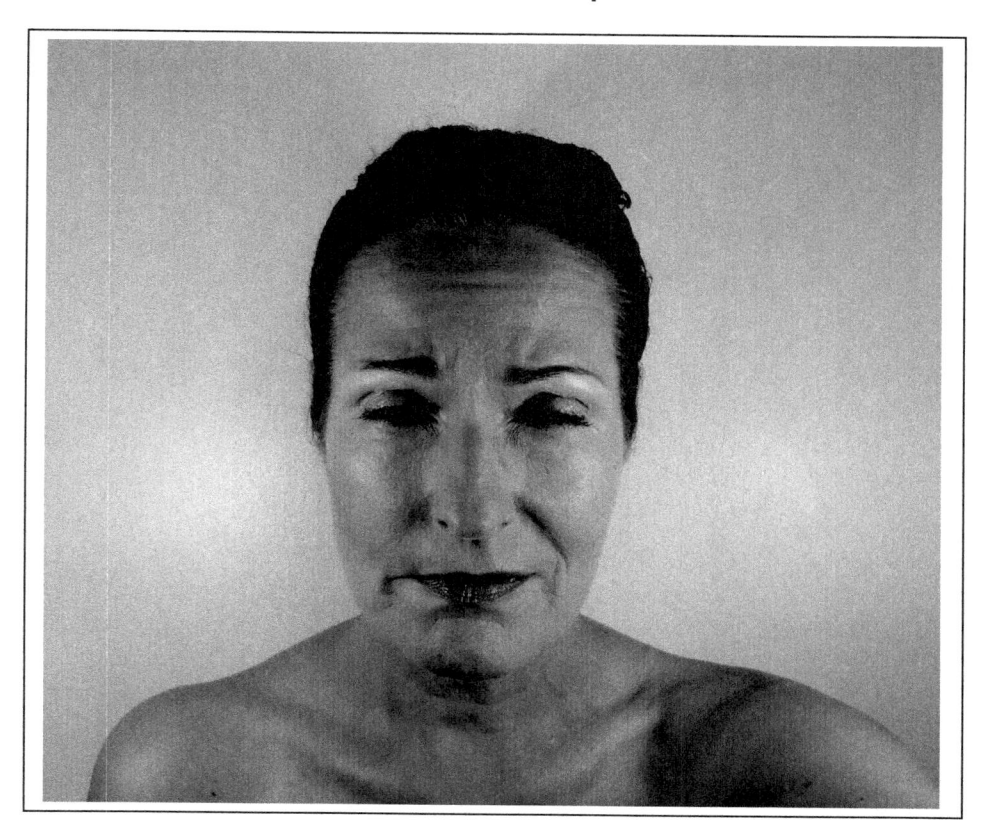

Scream with a big wide open mouth shaped like an "O" and raising your eyebrows high, opening out every muscle in your face pause, next
Screw up your whole face drawing in your eyebrows, shrivelling up your eyes and pulling your lips into a tight kiss, drawing in each and every facial muscle, pause.
Relax

Repeat 20 times

Note.
Your neck muscles will stand out and your décolletage will be lifted
Every facial muscle should come into play.

Exercises
WHOLE FACE 3
Scream n hold under eyes up

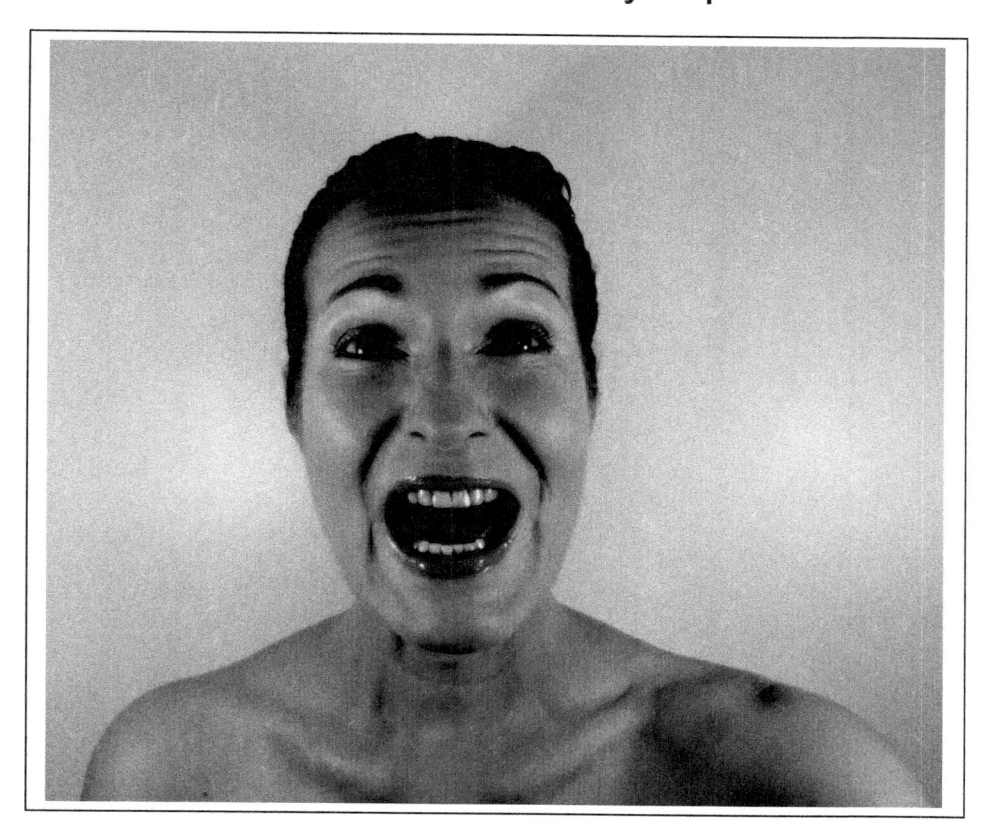

Scream with a big wide open mouth shaped like an "O" and raising your eyebrows high, opening out every muscle in your face pause,

Pull up your under eyelids, so high as to see your eyes are just slits

Hold: 1 minute

Note:
If it is too difficult for you, divide the exercise into two 30 second holds or even 4 x 15 second holds.

Exercises
WHOLE FACE 4
Whole face lift

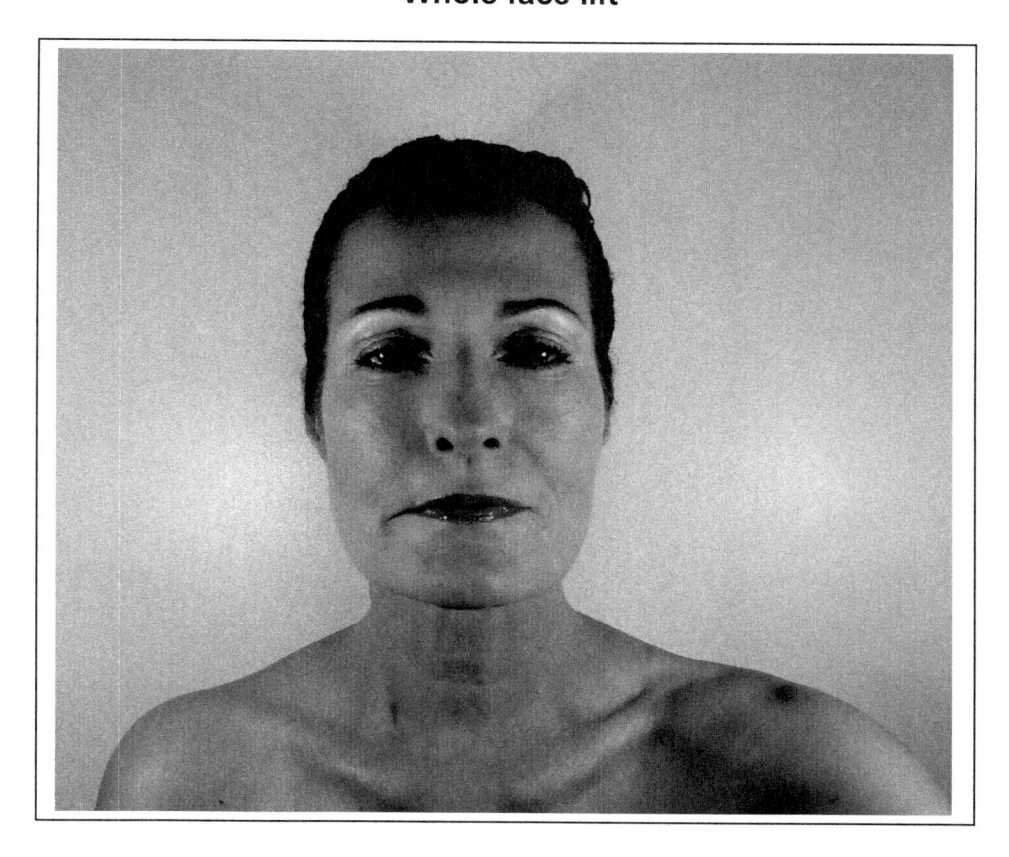

Teeth together, lips closed, tense every muscle in your face and neck. Eyebrows should be elevated fractionally and pulled out, a slight hint of a smile, flared nostrils, and pull in eye corners marginally pulled, under eyelid up and taut chin. It feels as if your whole face is being pulled back (as you will be exercising all the muscles that attach your face to the head and skull). You could even try to press your tongue into the roof of your mouth.

Hold: 1 minute **CONCENTRATE**

Note: This is singularly the most important exercise. There are no outwards visible signs of movement. **The only place I can even feel it externally is in front of my earlobes.**

Exercises
WHOLE FACE 5
Whole face taut

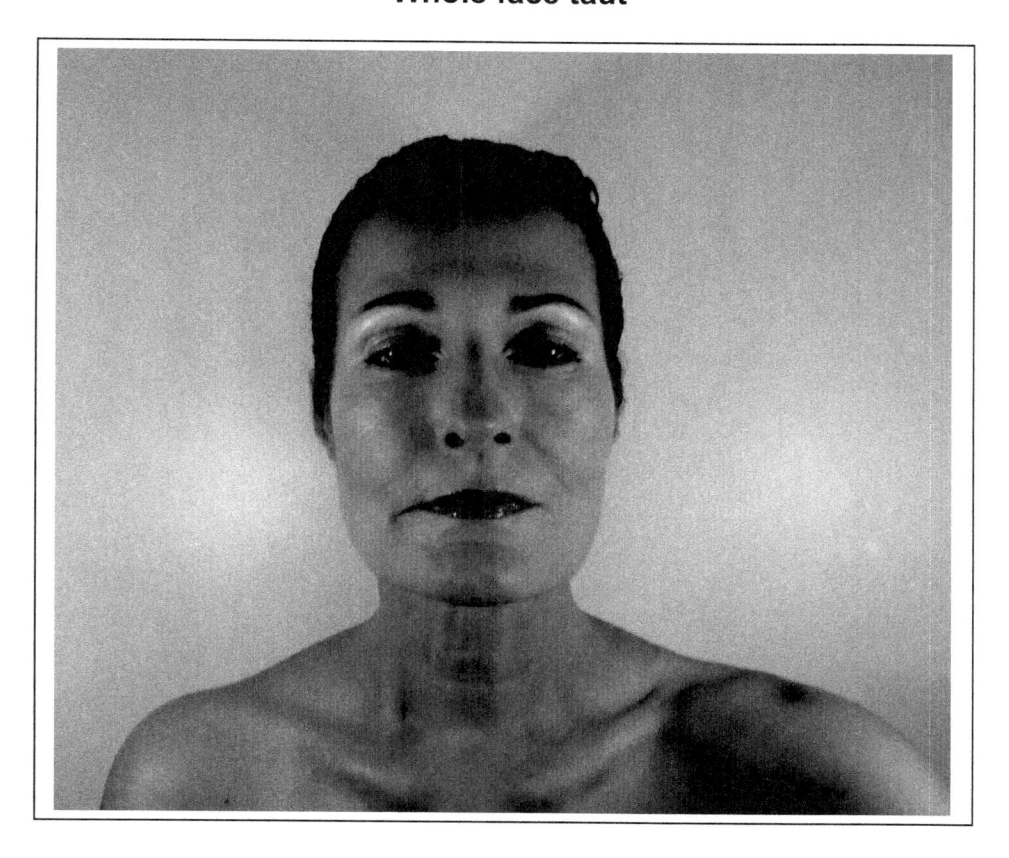

Teeth together, lips together with a subtle smile
Lift your eyebrows, up and out –hold fast
Lift your under eyelids up, until eyes are slits, preferably, so that the bottom lid touches the pupil (black circle in centre of the eye) then.
Smile as broadly as possible and then raise the corners of your mouth as high as possible to the corners of the eye.
Concentrate, make adjustments; but you may need to increase the eyebrow lift and or lift one side of the mouth more than the other
Hold: 1 minute
Note: This is an excellent exercise as a replacement for the 'whole face lift' if you are not able to accomplish that.

Exercises
WHOLE FACE 6
Your perfect face

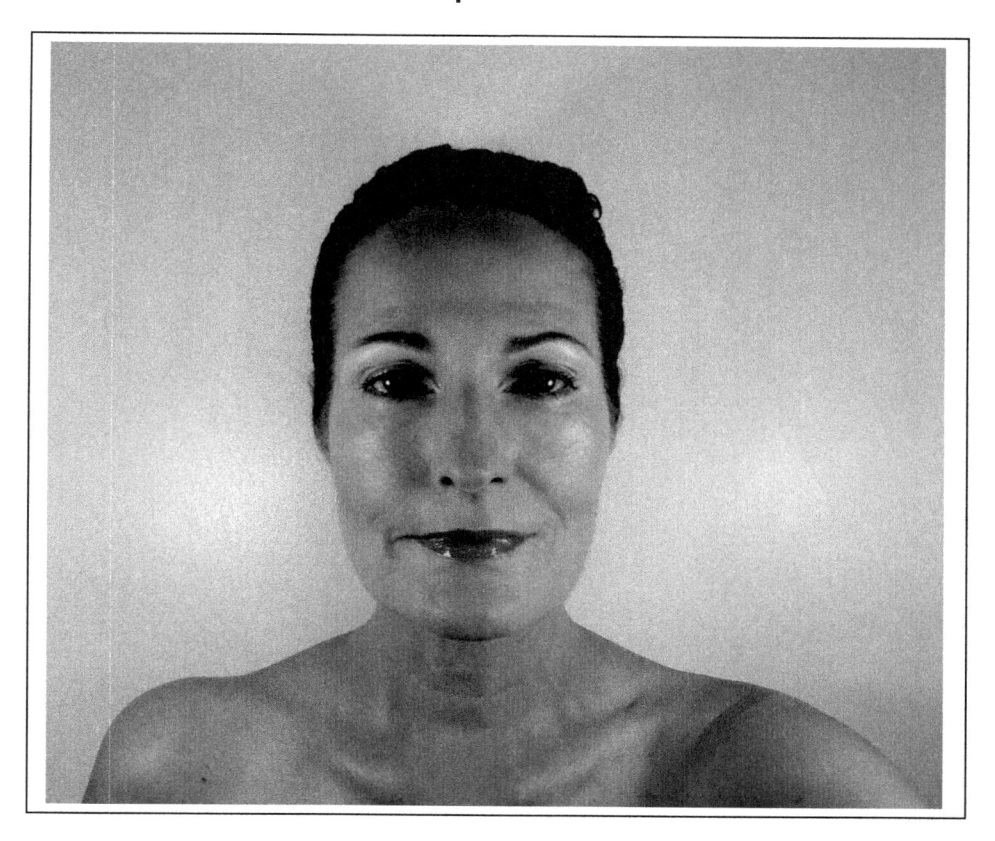

THE MOST ESSENTIAL EXERCISE FOR YOU
Look in the mirror, see what you don't like and change it!
Adjust your face to look the most attractive you can. Start by making the 'whole face facelift' and then adjust that face to **your perfect face**. **Concentrate** to teach all the muscles in the area to work together
Examples:
Frown – lift out back and up
Droopy smile –pull out and up
Neck –force tongue on to front teeth, clench neck muscles
Jowls –pull back the corners of the mouth from the ears and up to the temples
Remember: This is the face exercise to practice everywhere.

Exercises
MOUTH – Lower face 1
Mouth corners – smile n hold

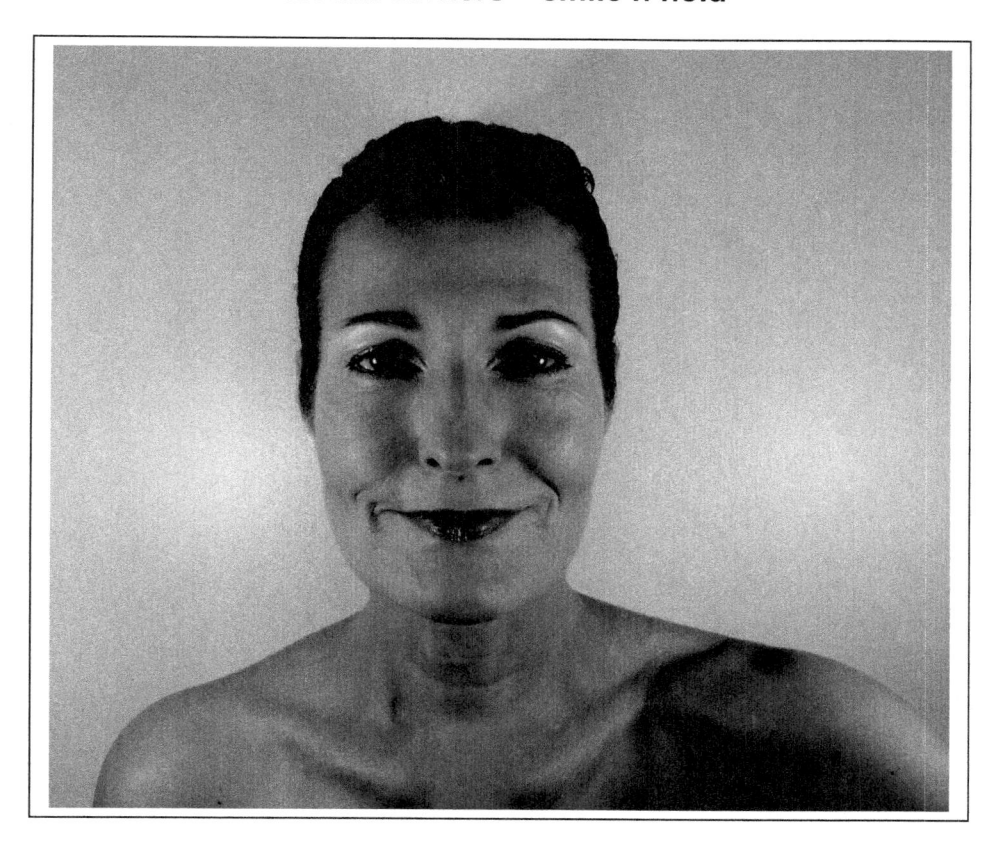

Lips and teeth together
Smile up to the corners of your eyes as far as you can (ensure corners are pointing upwards)
Make sure that your smile is even on both sides, if not adjust by lifting the corner to match the other one

Hold: 1 minute

Exercises
MOUTH – Lower face 2
Mouth corners –smile n kiss

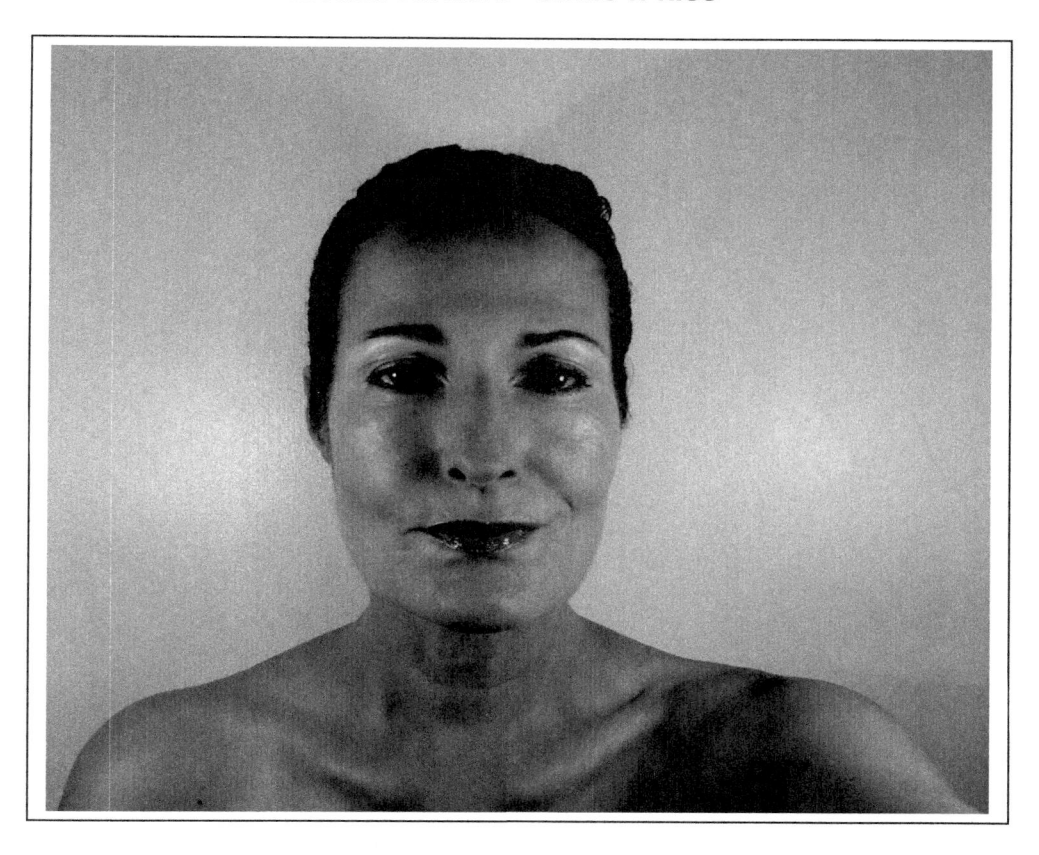

Teeth and lips together
Smile to your eye corners as high as possible, pause
Push your lips slowly forward into a kiss
Repeat continuously but very slowly in a fluid motion

Repeat: 15 times

Exercises
MOUTH – Lower face 3
Mouth corners – smile n cheeks up

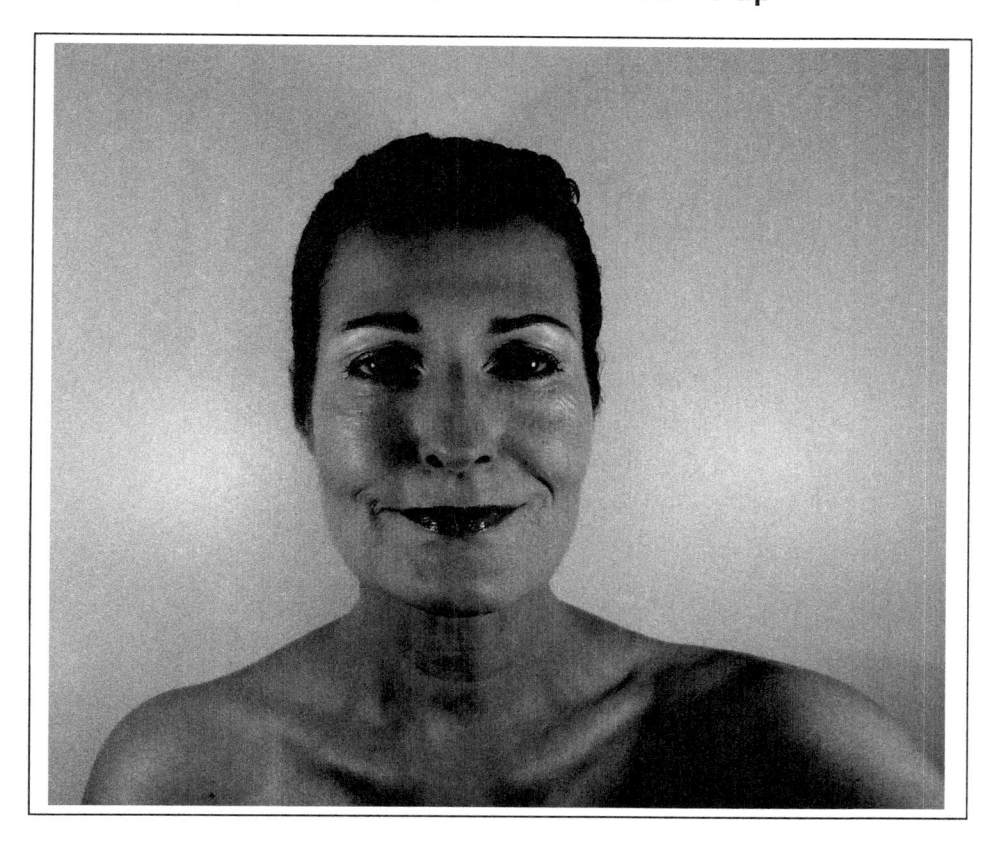

Teeth and lips together
Smile up to your eye corners as high as possible, pause

Pull up the corners of your eyes to lift cheeks up

Hold: 1 minute

Note:
It may help to also slightly lift the sides of your nose to engage the mouth to eye corner muscle. When you are experience, for a different feel, pull they eyebrows and corners of the nose in opposite directions.
For additional emphasis raise the chin to make dimples.

Exercises
MOUTH – Lower face 4
Chin - grin

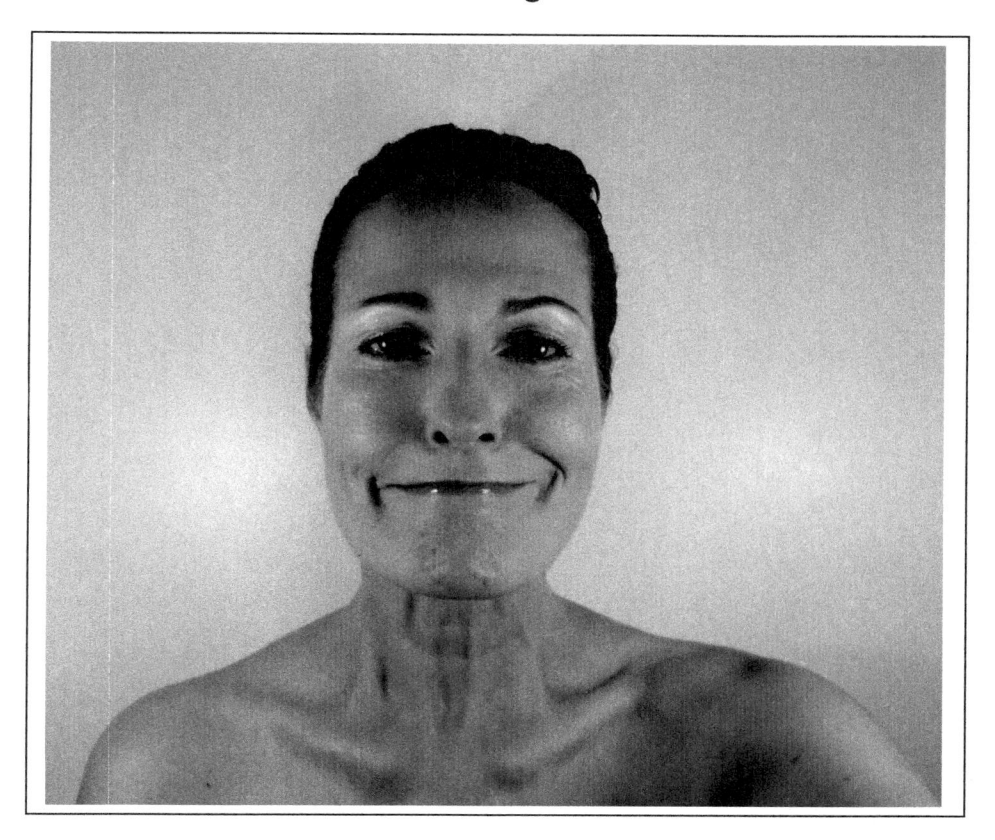

Lift up the muscles of your chin then
Smile, straight, pulling back towards your lower earlobes, a little, a little more in slow pulsing motions until your smile is very pulled back

Lift up your cheeks to the corners of your eyes then

Hold: 1 minute

Note:
Keep pulling a straight smile back and adjust as necessary throughout.

Exercises
MOUTH – Lower face 5
Chin - Hard grin

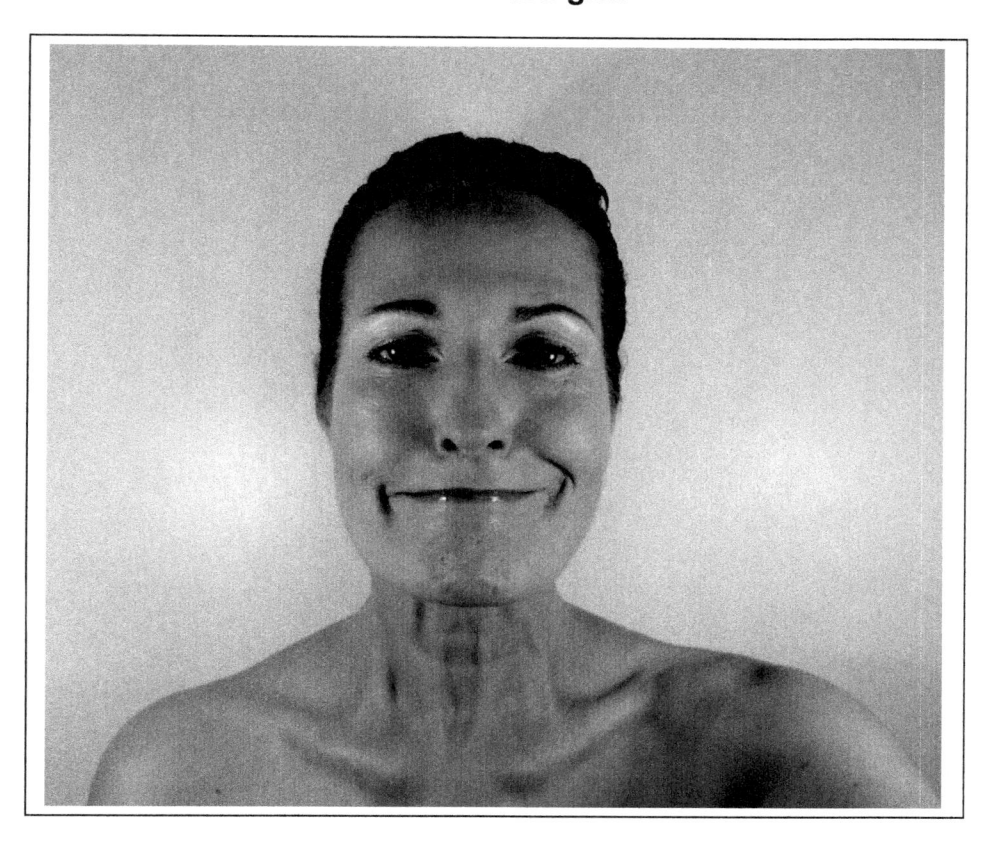

Teeth and lips together
Pull your mouth very wide but straight
Press your lips tightly together (they may want to form a kiss – don't let them. The edges may also want to turn down, don't let them – keep level by forcing your mouth upwards) and

Hold: 1 minute

Exercises
MOUTH – Lower face 6
Chin – Tongue press

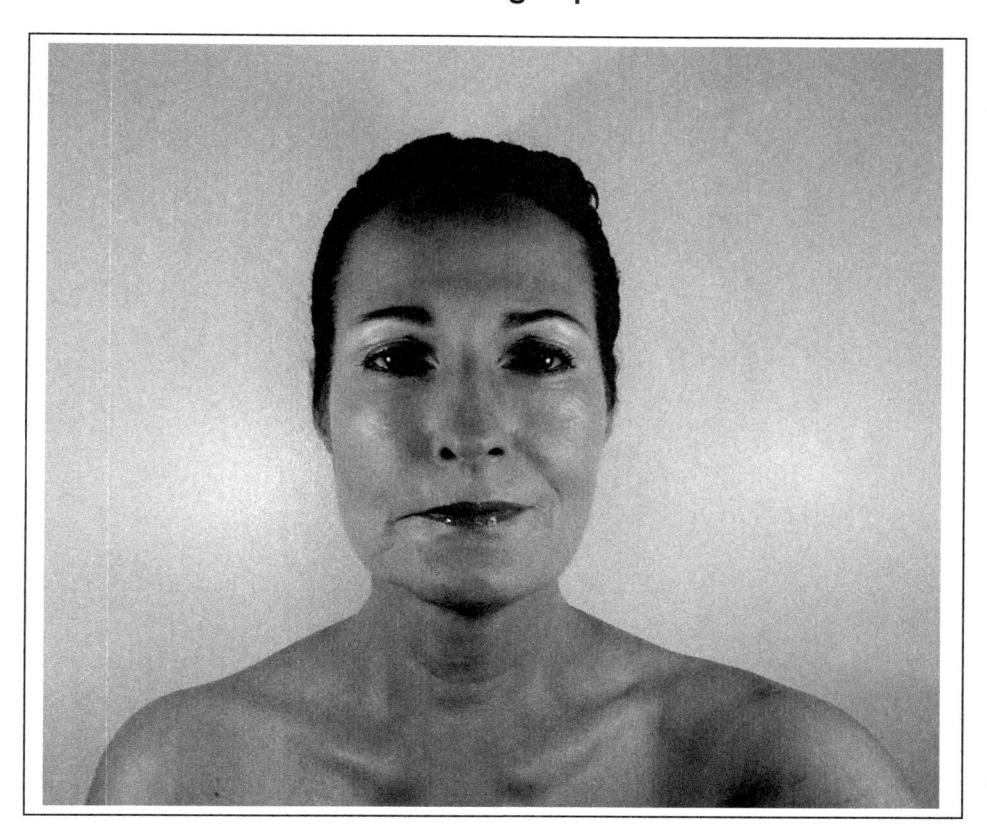

Teeth and lips together
Press your tongue hard into the roof of your mouth and

Hold: 1 minute

Note:
You may need to swallow or relax your push, if so just do so and start again
See how under the chin becomes pushed out.

Exercises
EYES - 1
Bags up

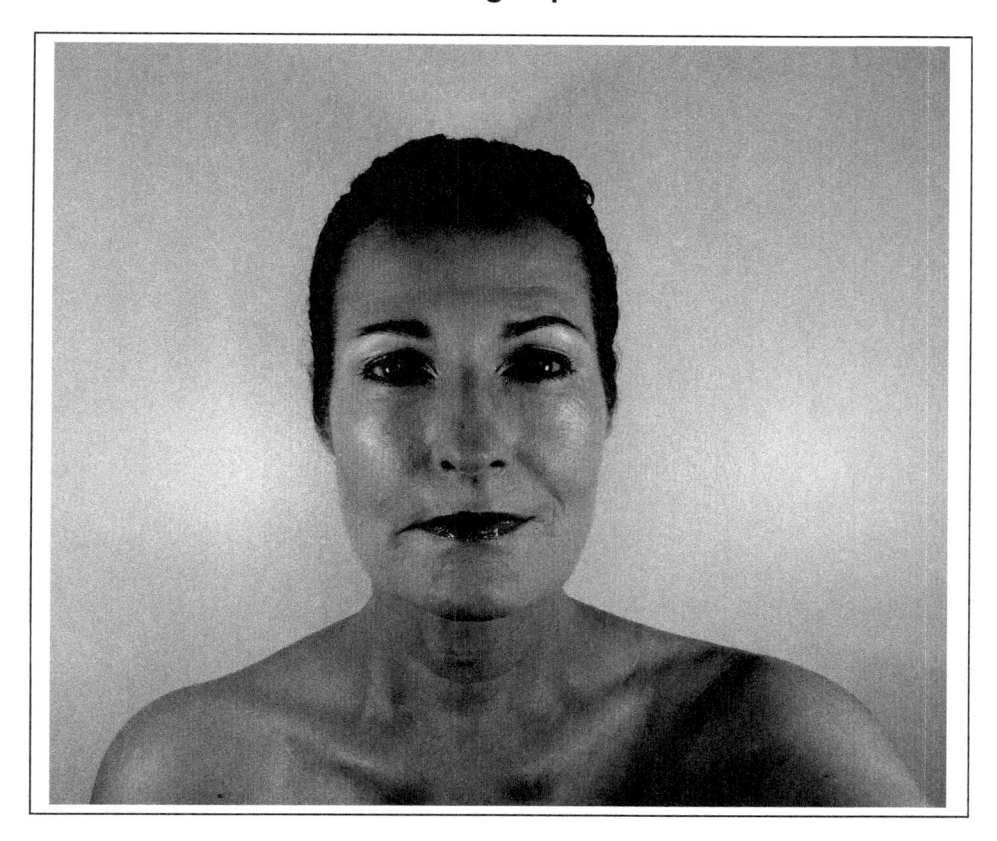

Pull your under eyelids up and

Hold; 1 minute

You may prefer and find it easier to lift and relax the under eye continuously for 50 times

Note:
Try to also pull the eyes out towards the temples and keep the eyes wide open but the eyebrows relaxed.

**Exercises
EYES - 2
Ultra stares**

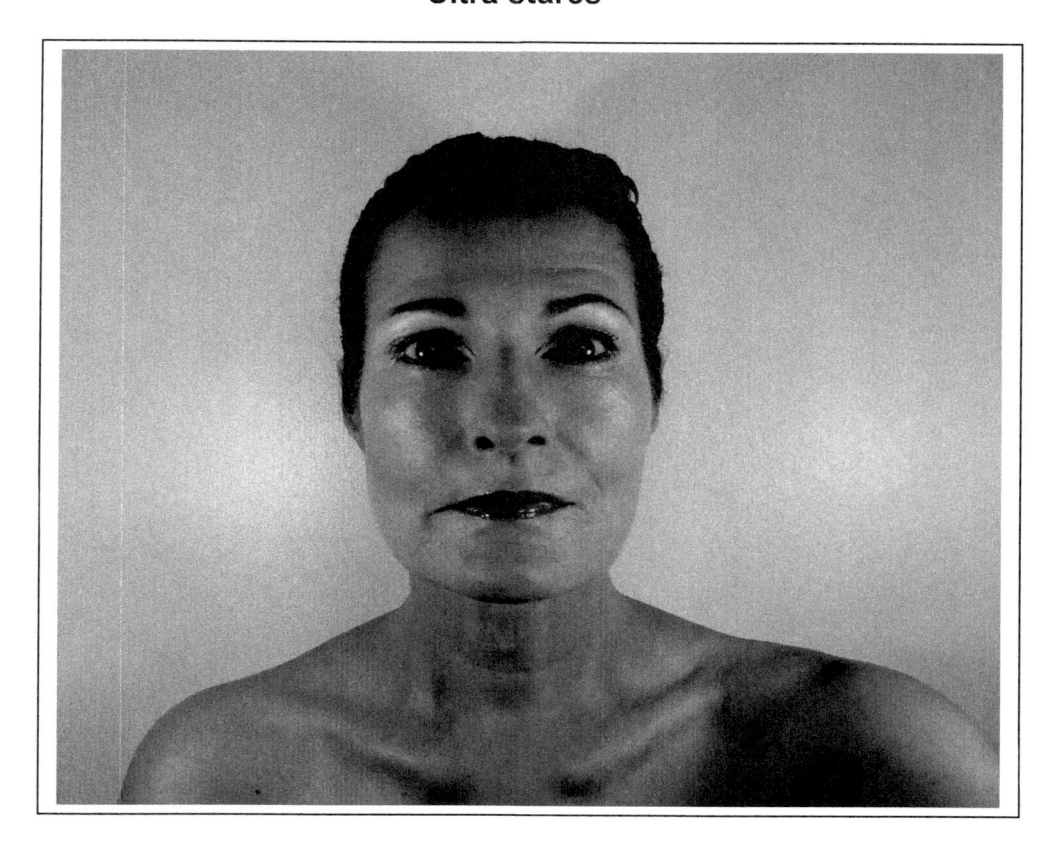

Locate a spec about 2 feet to a yard/meter in front of you, maybe on your mirror or your computer screen.

Focus on the spot and stare. Hold the stare as long as you can without blinking. Your eyes will widen, your eyebrows will move up. When you cannot hold it any longer relax and start again.

Hold: 1 minute

Exercises
EYES - 3
Eye circles

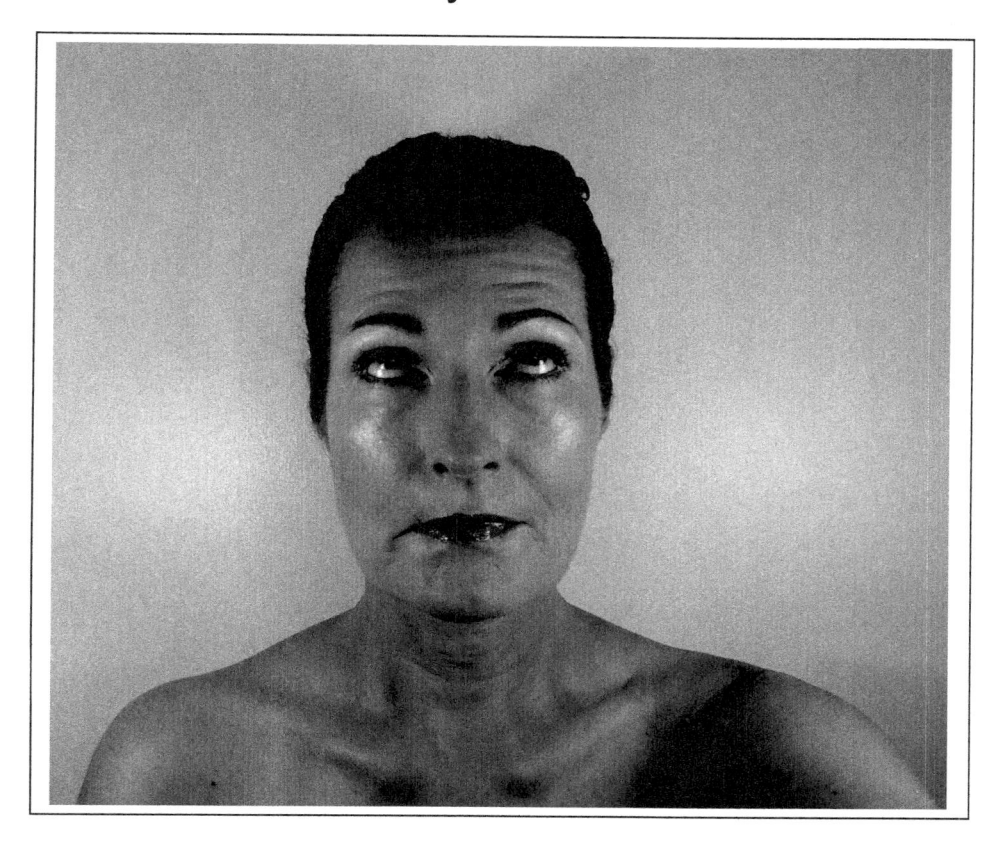

Look up as far as possible, roll down to the left side as far as possible; continue in a downward circular motion to the bottom and roll up to the right, continuing up to the top to complete the circle.

Repeat 3 times in total
Reverse

Repeat 3 times

Exercises
EYES - 4
Eyes in and out

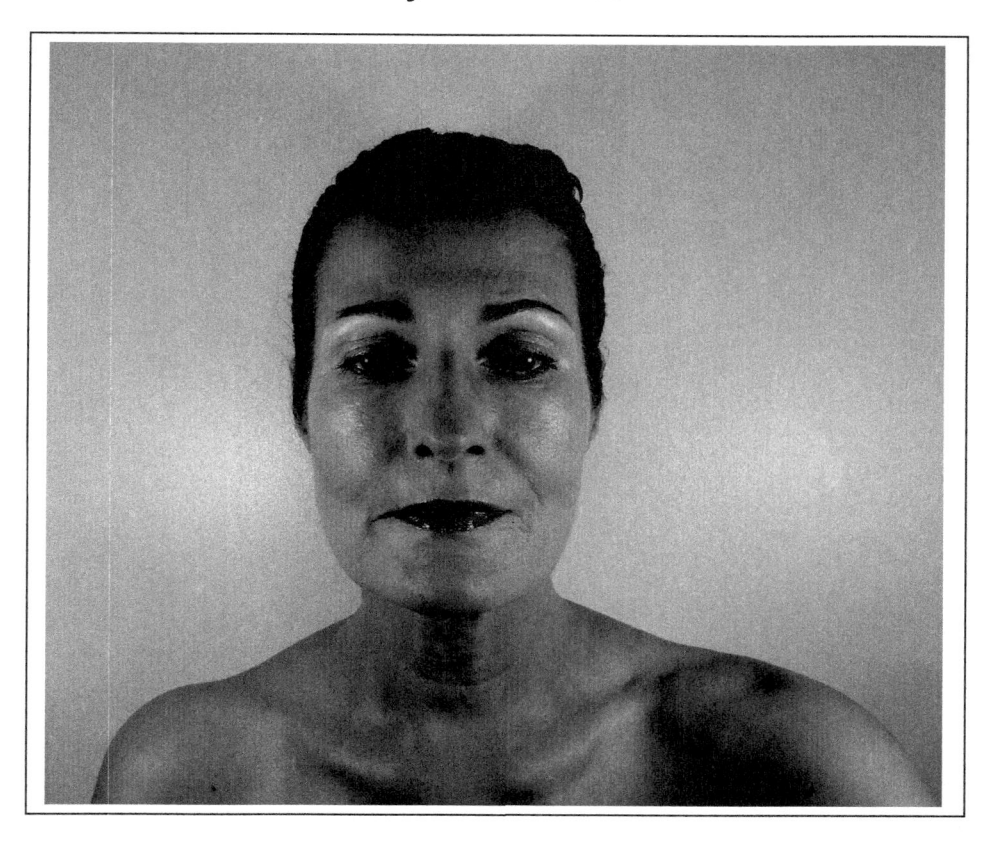

With eyes open naturally wide
Draw your eyes into the bridge of the nose slowly
Pause
Draw your eyes out towards the temples on either side of the face
Pause

Repeat 10 times

Note;
It is difficult when pulling the eyes out, it may help you, if at the pause you to try to think of looking behind you simultaneously on both sides. This is of course impossible!

**Exercises
EYES - 5
Winks**

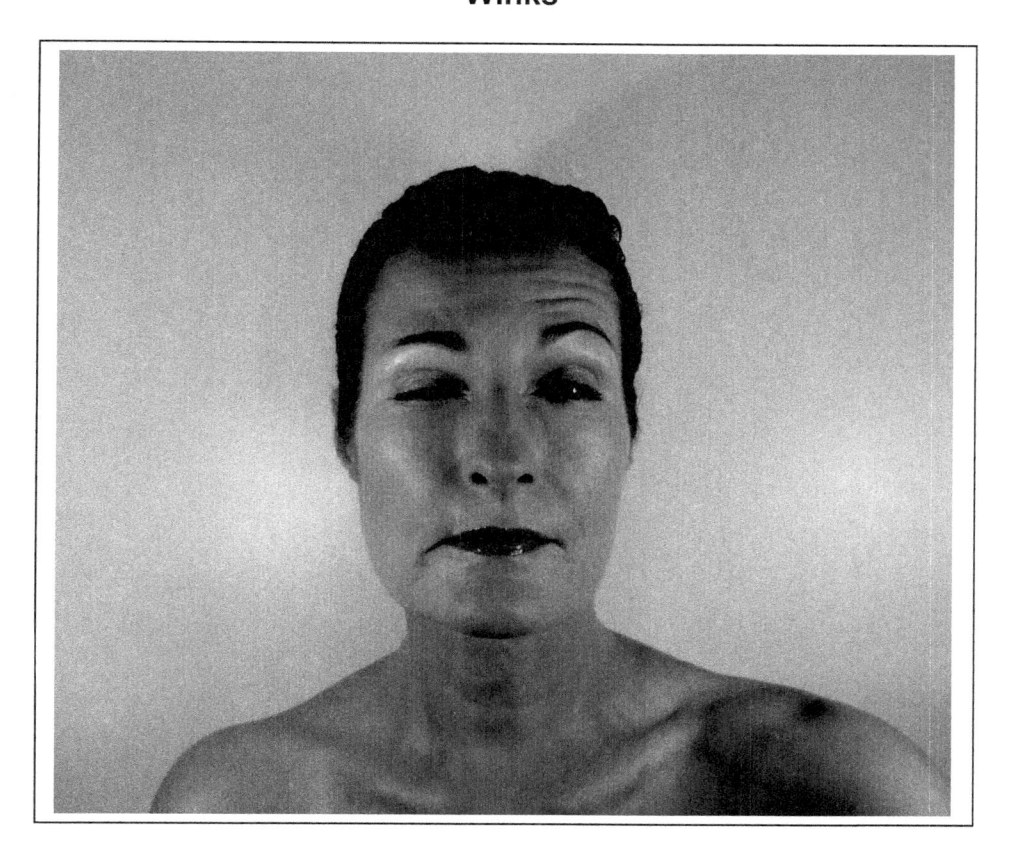

Shut one eye, while keeping the other eye open.
(Try to fully open the other with a raised eyebrow)
Pause and hold

Repeat: 3 times on each eye

Note:
Form is more important than number of repetitions achieved
Really try to open the eye as wide as possible

We are not all made the same as discussed earlier and I find this very difficult, hence I'm not keen on it, hence the muscle isn't strengthened!

Exercises
EYES - 6
Eye pulls

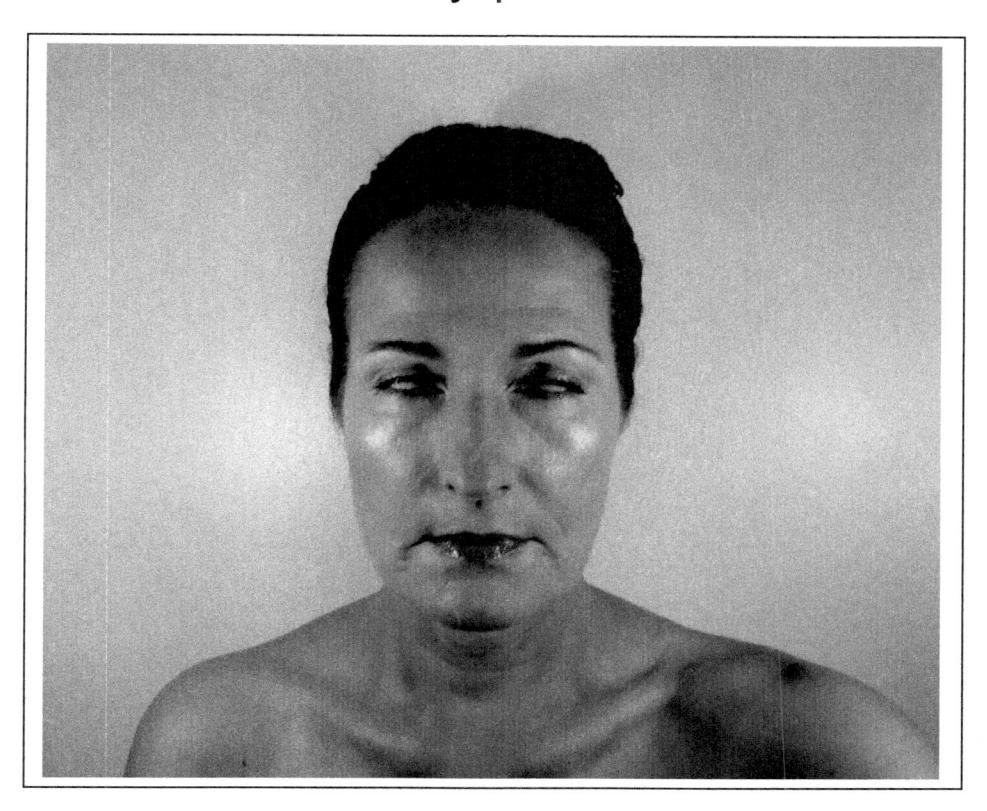

Look in the mirror
Pull up the under eyelids until you can hardly see out and your eyes, look like slits, next
Raise eyebrows high, keep them lifted throughout then
Gradually, very, very slowly release the tension on you upper eyelid and open fully until you are staring
Release

Note:
Ideally this should take a minute, but start with whatever suits you, 20 seconds or 30 seconds and adjust repetitions to suit 1 minute.

**Exercises
MOUTH – Upper 1
Nasolabial folds – tongue holds**

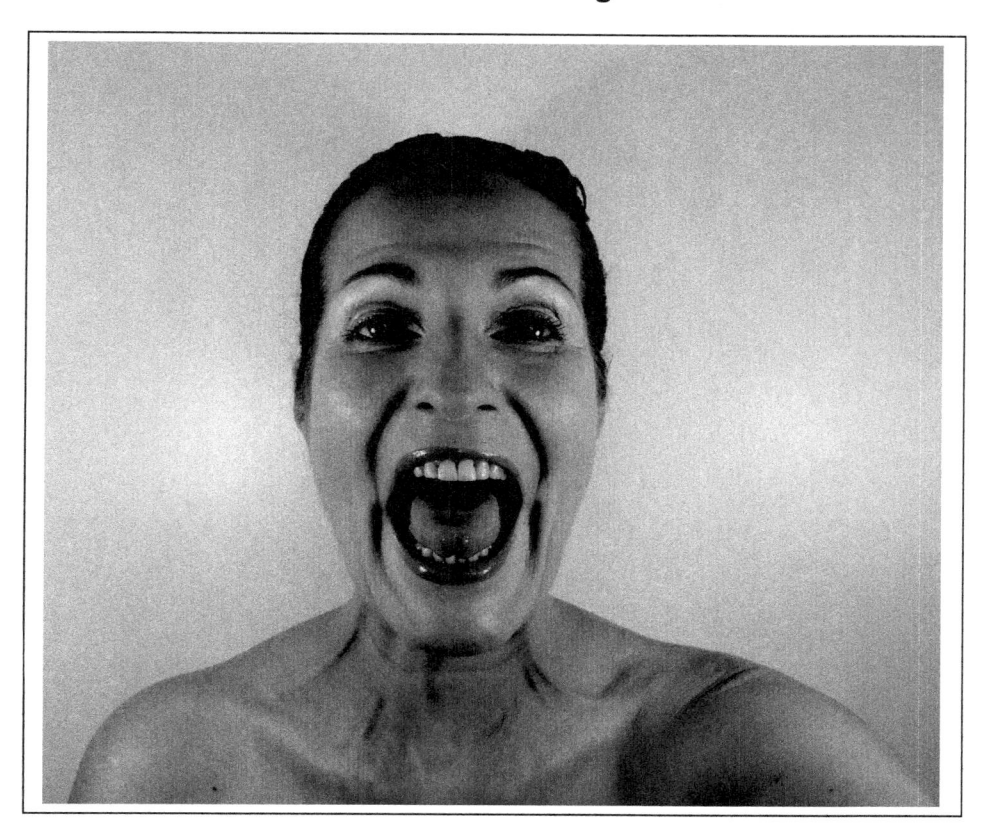

Stick your tongue out as far as possible and

Hold: 1 minute

Note:
For an extra pull, lift your eyebrows and even more advanced lift your under eyes.

For an extra pull on the neck, curl your tongue into the back of your upper teeth and press.

However, it is more productive to do the first part correctly than add the extensions and only be able to hold the pose for 30 seconds.

Exercises
MOUTH – Upper 2
Nasolabial folds - tongue sides in n out

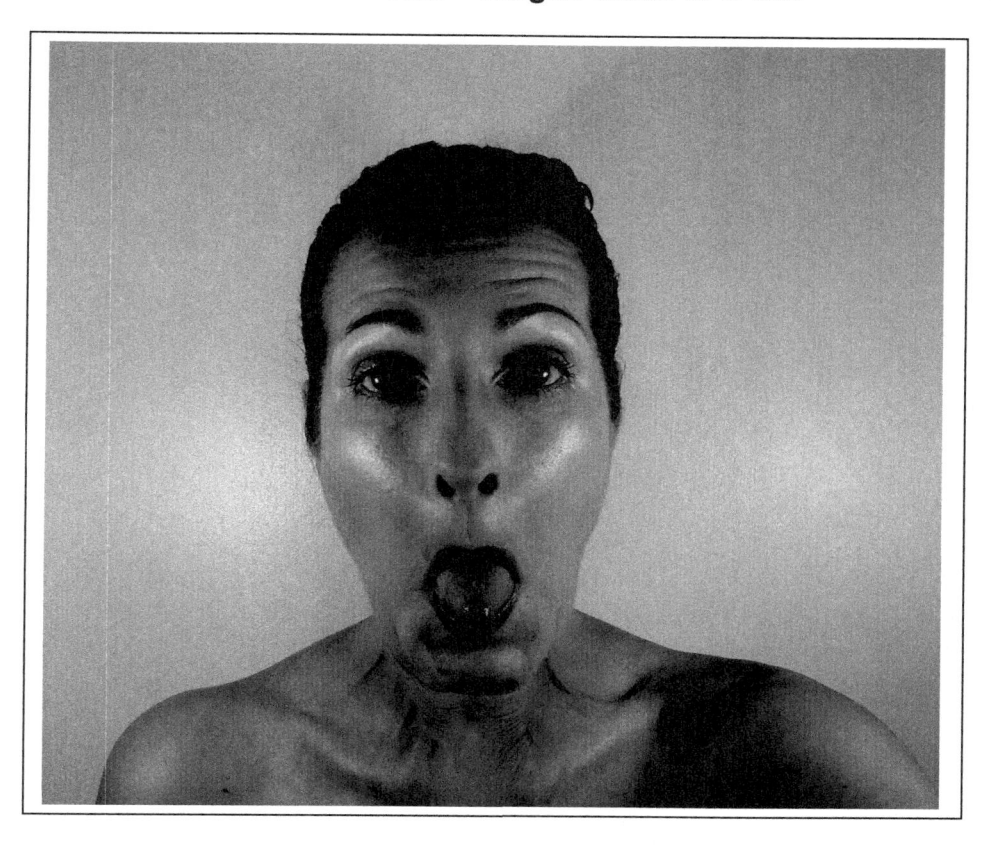

Stick your tongue out as far as possible

Bring in the sides of your mouth slowly then
Release them slowly back outwards
Repeat bringing the sides of your mouth in and out 5 times
Relax

Repeat 3 times

Note:
Your neck muscles should be standing and your eyebrows should be raised naturally. For a real additional pull when you are an experienced practitioner you may also care to lift your under eyelids, however form is most important.

Exercises
MOUTH – Upper 3
Nasolabial folds – surprised snarl

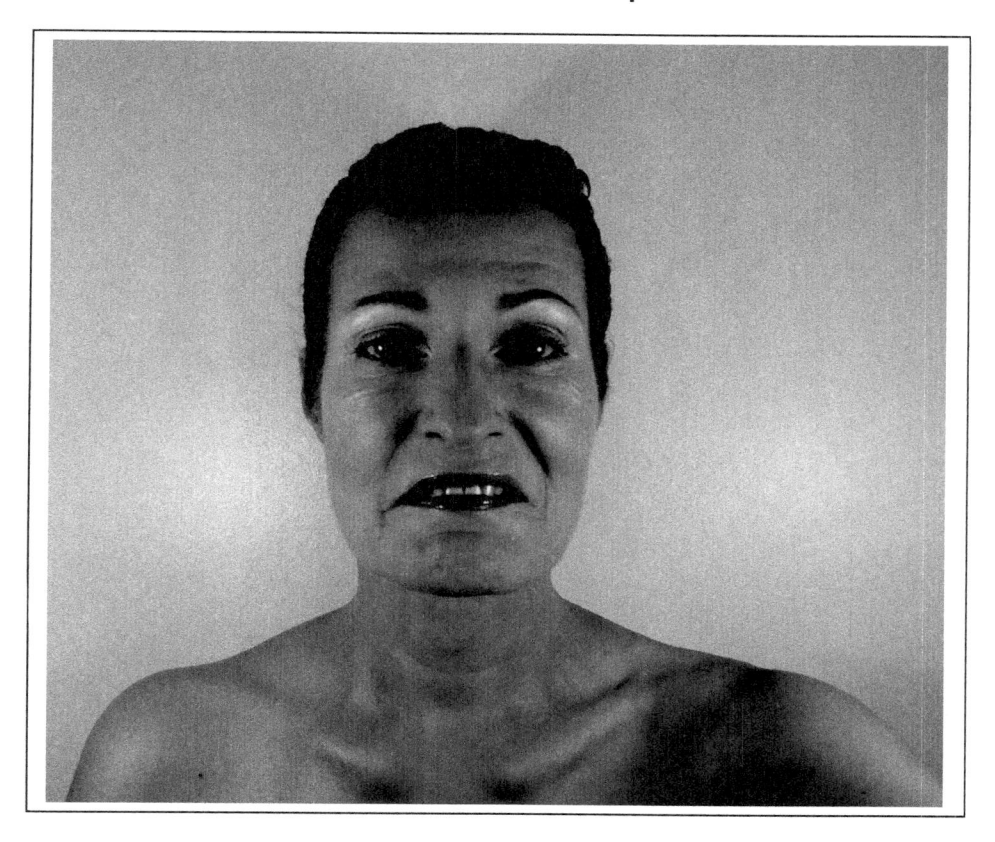

Teeth together and lips closed
Draw up front lip into a snarl, next
Pull up forehead by moving muscle between eyebrows
Then make a wide, a very smile, trying to turn the corners of the mouth upward then
Pull chin down and

Hold: 1 minute

Exercises
MOUTH – Upper 4
Cheeks - smiles

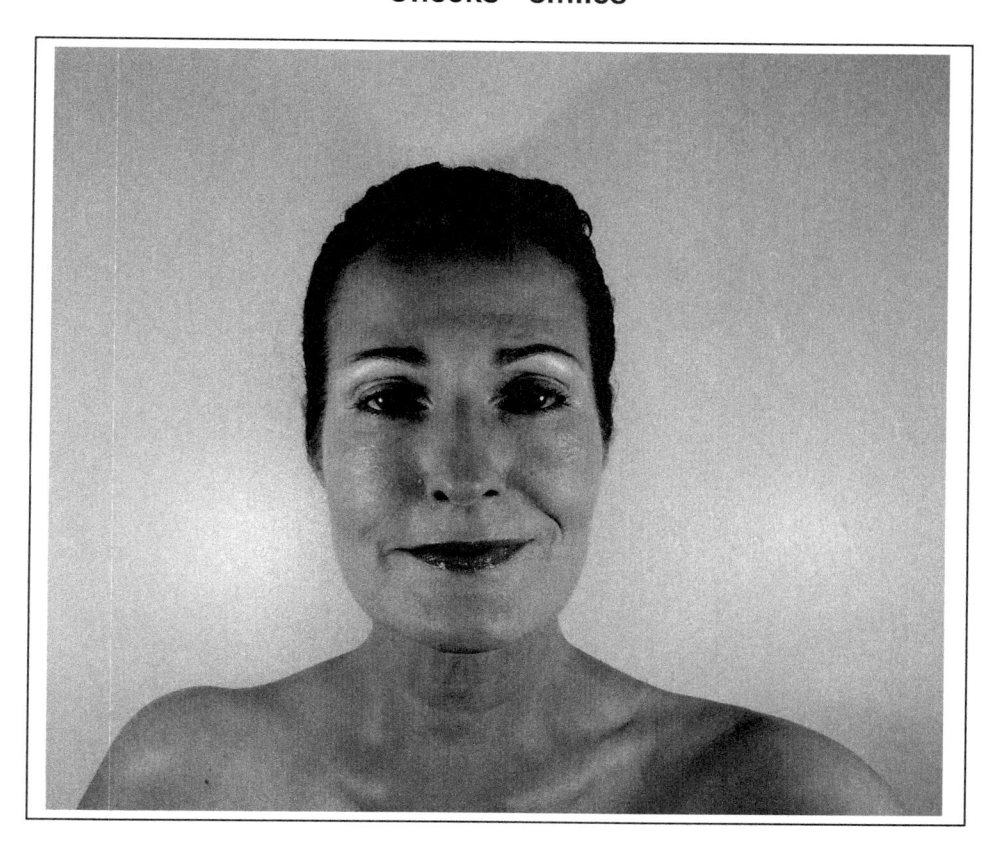

Teeth together lips barely touching
Smile
Wide, wider, widest, turning up the mouth corners then
Make mini pulling backwards movements
Pulling back slightly more each time
Do not relax, pull back 50 times

Note:
This is hard if you are doing it correctly and you will see your cheekbones rise and fall. For an additional difficulty try raising your eyebrows in synchronisation with your cheeks.

Exercises
MOUTH – Upper 5
Cheeks – open smile to whistle

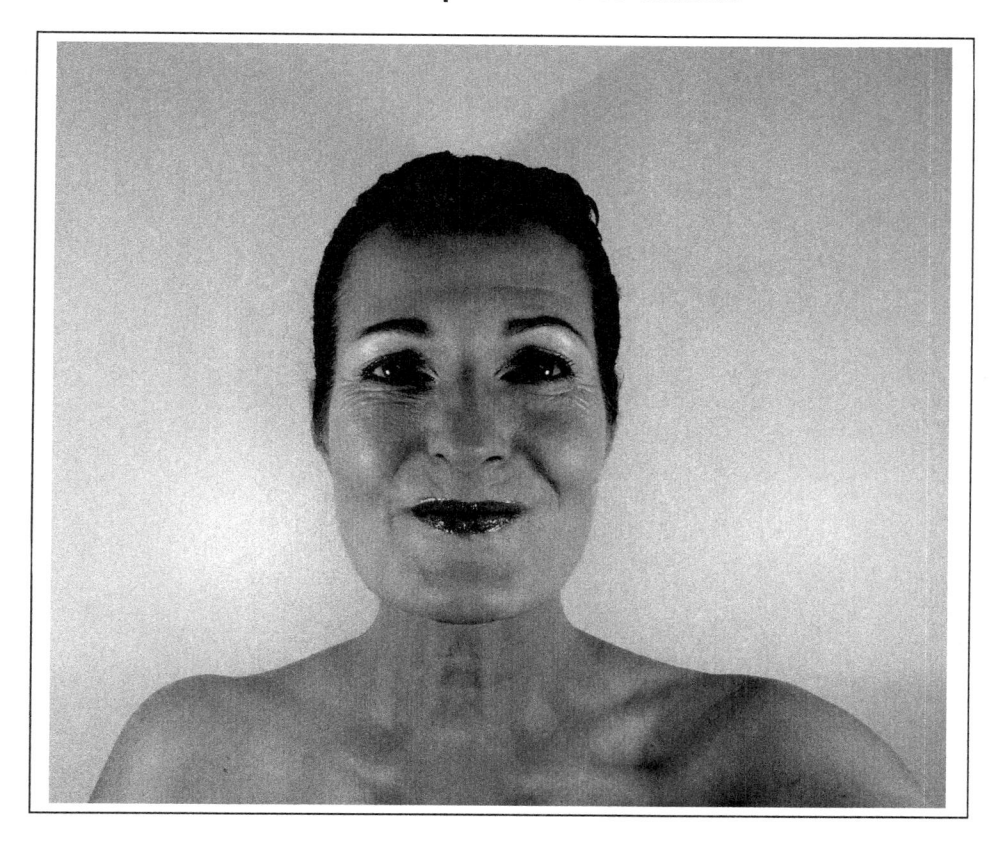

Teeth together, lips together
Smile wide up to corners of the eye as far as possible then
Relax a little to slowly draw lips forward into a whistle, next
Relax a little to slowly draw lips out and up at the corners and
Relax a little to slowly draw lips forward into a whistle

Repeat 5 times

Note:
This is a fluid continuous motion. It is easy to fake it by doing it fast, slowly is what counts – maintaining a smile and lips closed until the whistle.

Exercises
MOUTH – Upper 6
Cheeks – open smile n cheeks up

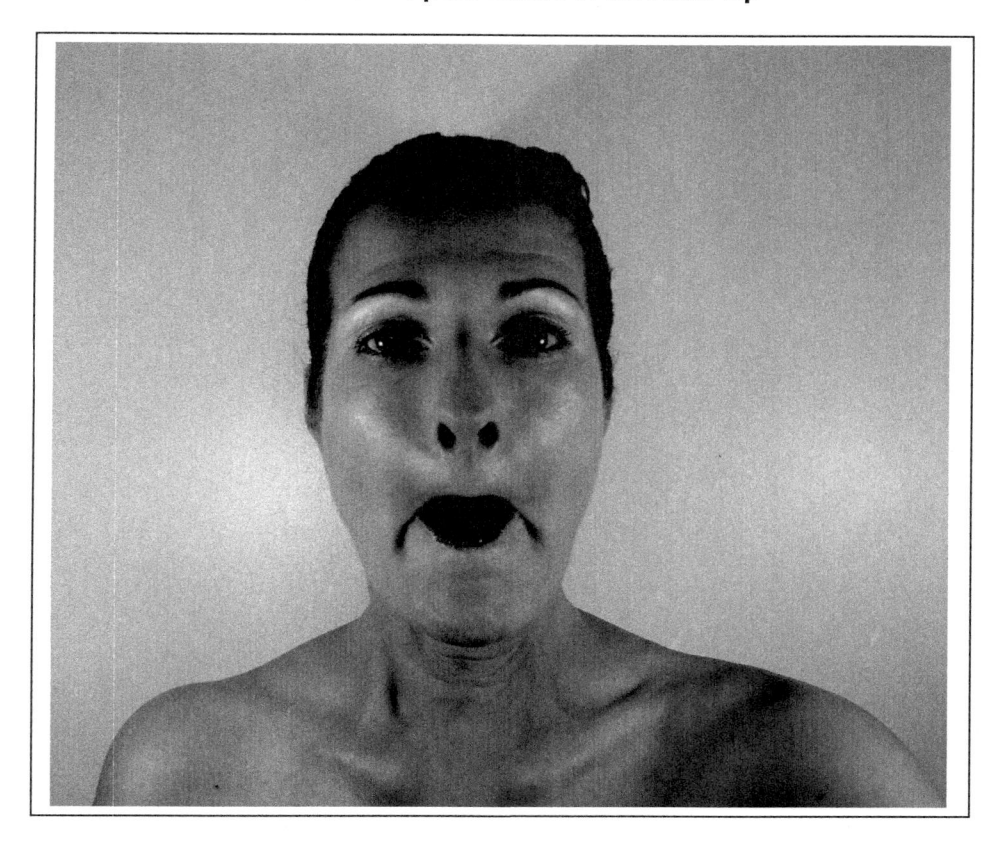

Teeth together
Open your mouth very wide with your lips pulled up back over gums

Pull lips back as far and as wide as you can then

Hold: 1 minute

Note:
For an increased pull, pull up they under eyelids. And even more advanced pull up and out the eyebrows.

Exercises
NECK - 1
Sad face jowls

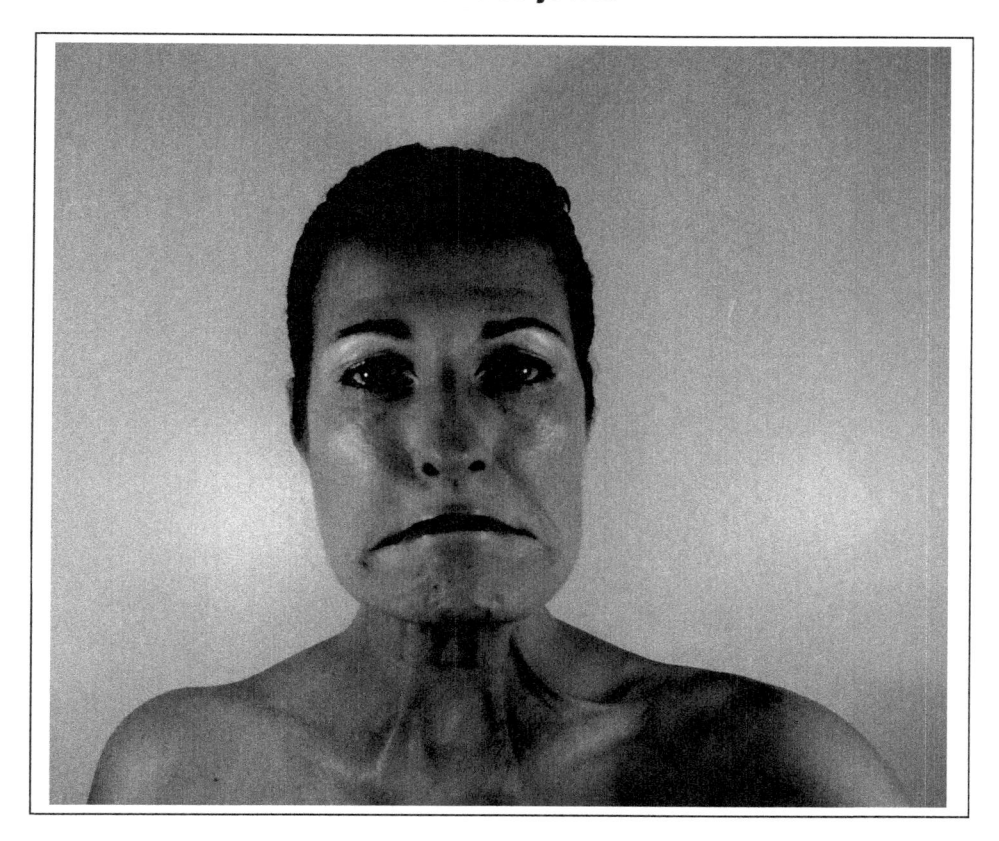

Teeth together, lips together.

Pull down the corners of both sides of the mouth
(The lower lip and neck muscles will be flexed) next
Draw up chin (which will dimple) then
Pull left mouth corner and hold - 5 seconds
Pull right mouth corner hold - 5 seconds
Pull back equally on each side - straight back to make something like a dimple
Keep the neck and chin tense
Hold for 45 seconds
Bonus a fuller bottom lip.

Exercises
NECK - 2
Nods

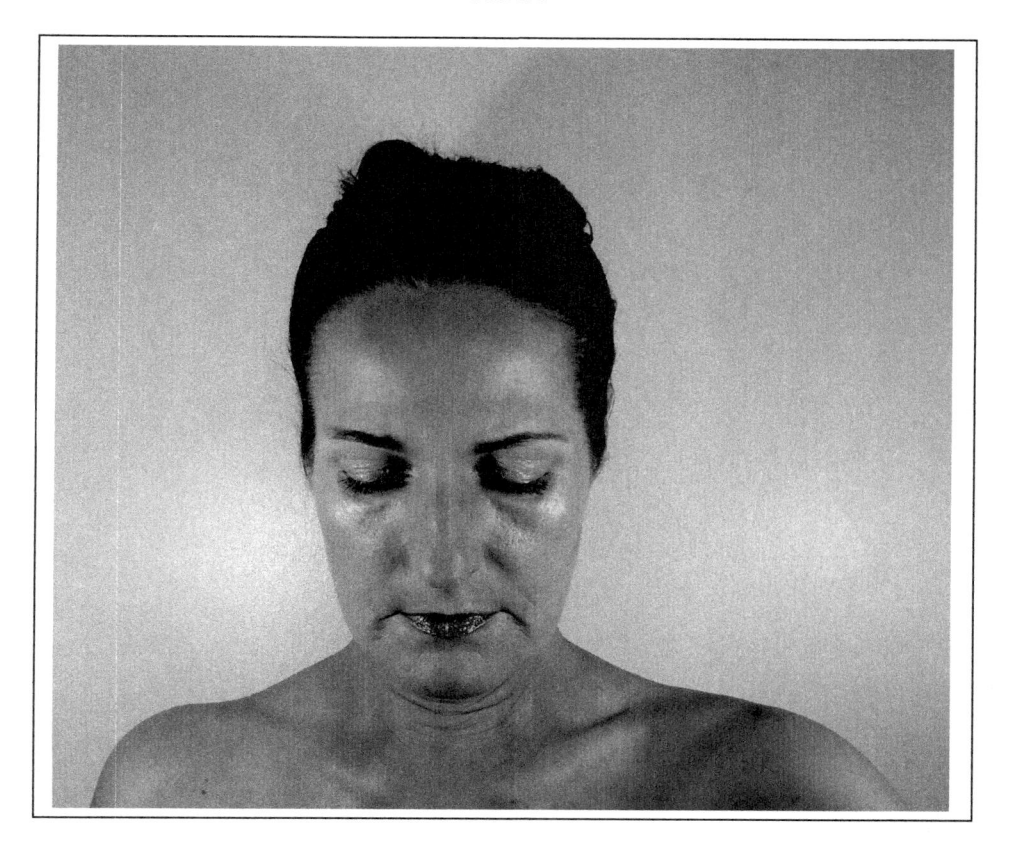

Teeth and lips together

Drop your head forwards only to its' natural position then
Make five little nods, afterwards
Bring your head back to an upright position

Repeat 5 times

Stretches back of neck
Relaxing

Exercises
NECK - 3
Back kisses

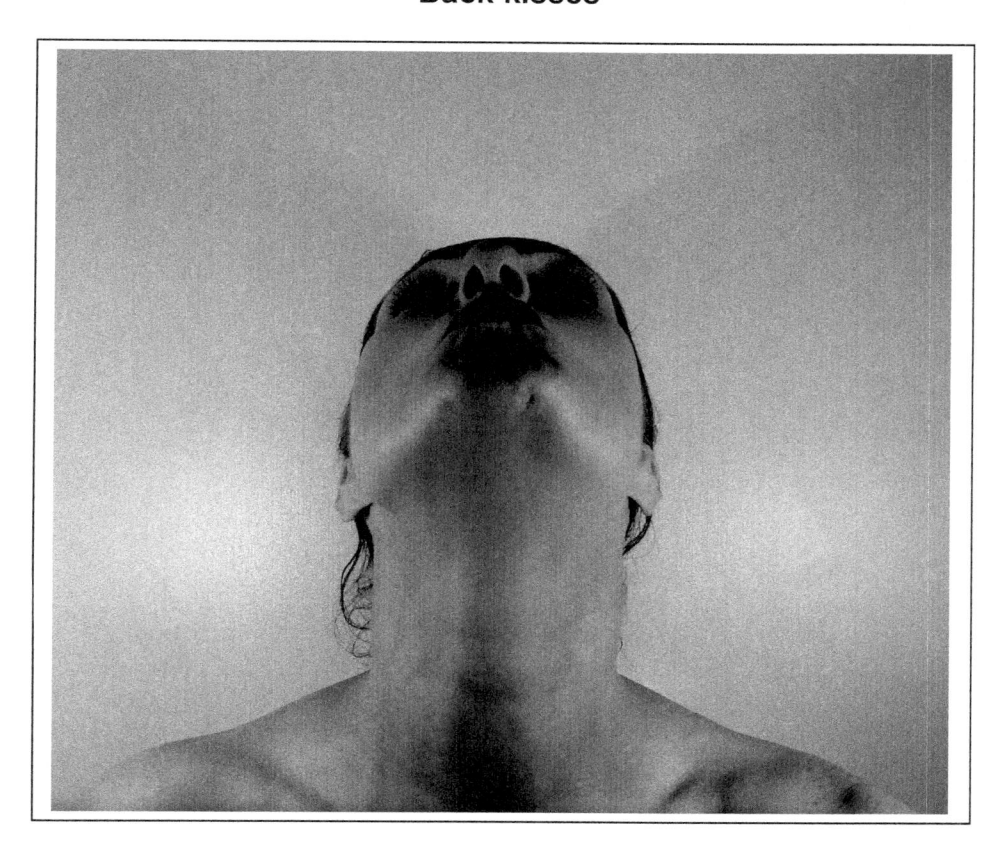

Teeth and lips together

Slowly look up and drop your head backwards to look at the ceiling, then
Bring your jaw forward, purse lips into a kiss and slowly kiss the ceiling 5 times
Slowly bring the head forward to neutral

Repeat 4 times

Exercises
NECK - 4
Side flops

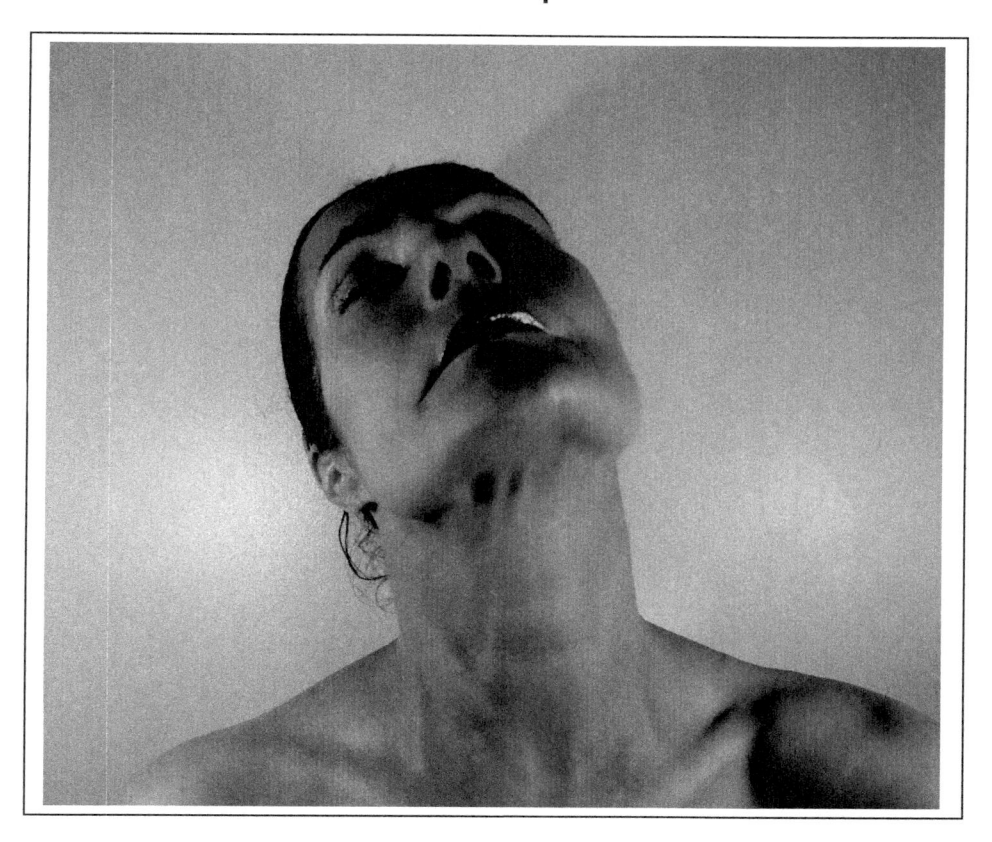

Teeth and lips together

Flop your head forwards, then
Slowly lift your head and, look to the ceiling. Gently flop your head to the left bring your head back upright and look to the ceiling and gently flop your head to the right.

Repeat flopping side to side for 5 times each side
Bring your head back to the centre and repeat again

Note:
Keep your shoulders relaxed.

Exercises
NECK - 5
Twists

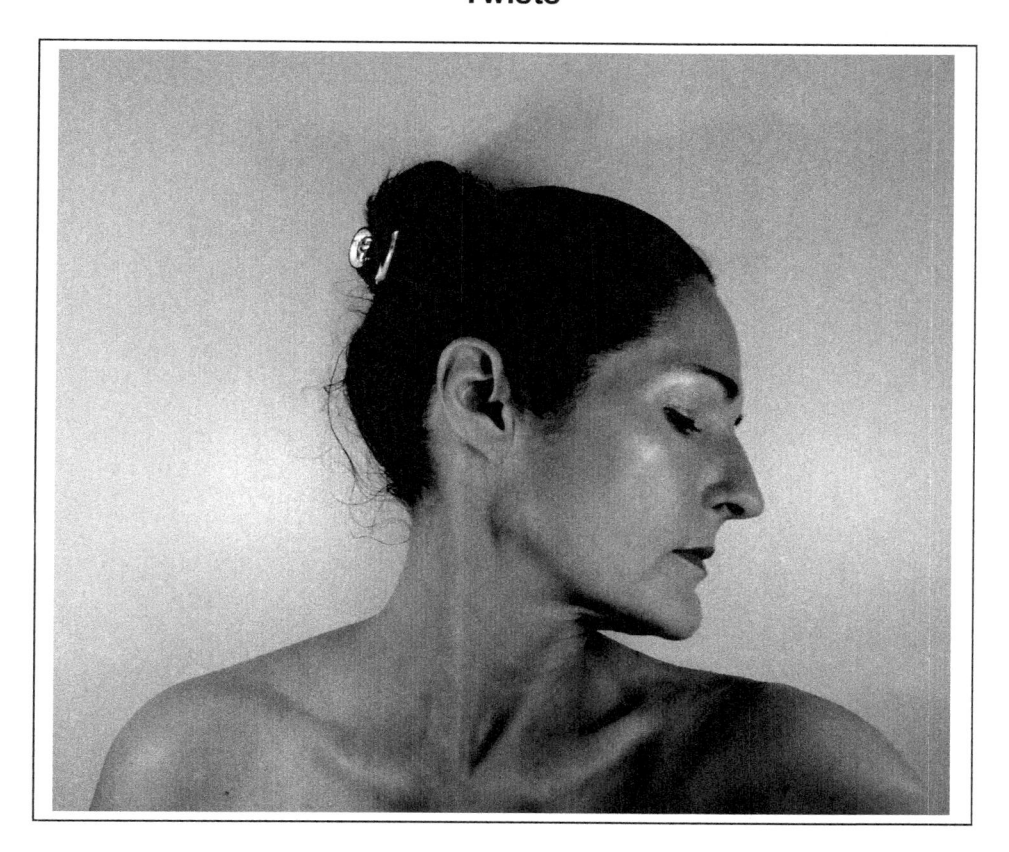

Teeth and lips together and face facing forwards

With your chin down close to your chest
Turn left, pause turn right, then back to centre
Repeat 5 times (5 each side)

With your chin level
Turn left, pause turn right, then back to centre
Repeat 5 times (5 each side)

With your chin facing the ceiling
Turn left, pause turn right, then back to centre
Repeat 5 times (5 each side)

Exercises
NECK - 6
Décolletage pull ups

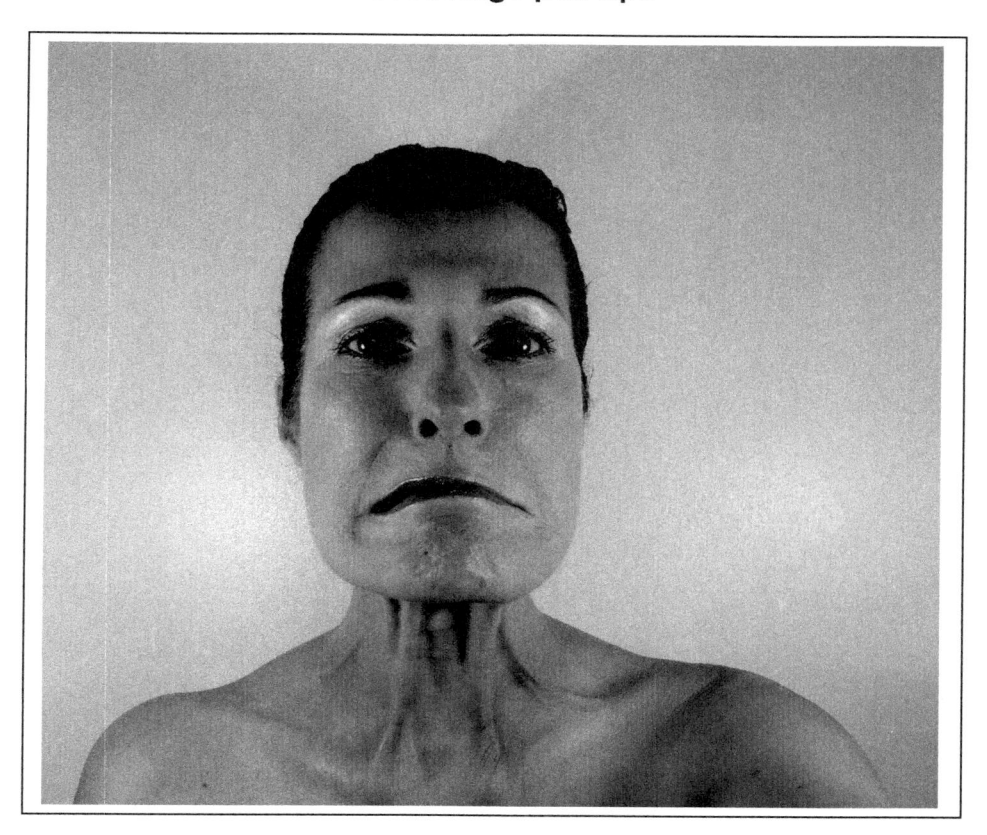

Teeth together, lips parted

First pull lips down
Then pull back corners of your mouth as far as you can, flex your neck muscles; this will bring up the décolletage. Keep pulling back.

Hold 10 seconds, relax

Repeat 5 times

Note:
You may also feel this in your upper cheek area.
This exercise also makes a fuller bottom lip.

Cool Down
1
Ear rubs

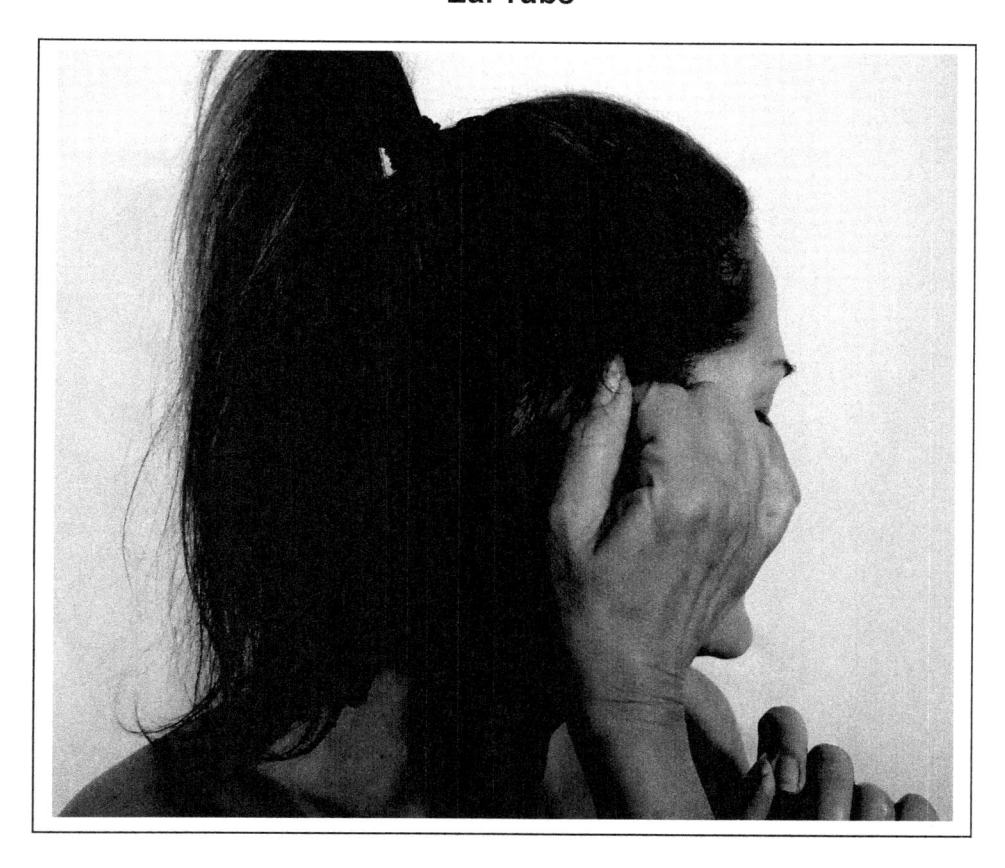

Put each of your index fingers in your ear holes and
Place each of your thumbs behind your ear lobes then
Move the fingers around in the ear holes, while rubbing behind each ear, moving to the top of each

Reverse your finger position at the top then
Pinch and rub outer ear on the way down

Note:
This is an uncomplicated movement of massaging the ears to suit what makes you happy, soft and slow or hard and fast.

Cool Down
2
Hair pulls

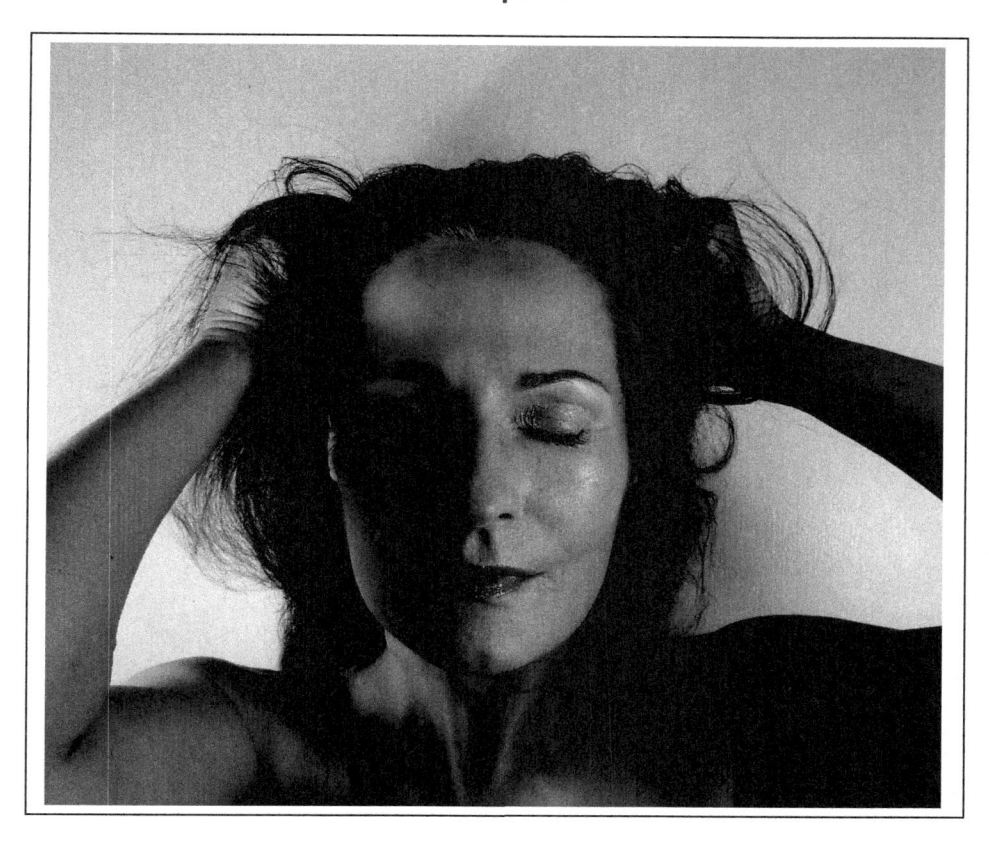

With the fingers on both hands grab some of your hair in front of your ears. Make circular motions, 3 times in each direction
Move the hands up to the temples and make circular motions, 3 times in each direction next
Move the hands up an inch and make circular motions, 3 times in each direction then
Move fingers about your ear and make circular motions, 3 times in each direction afterwards
Keep making hair pull circles throughout your hair
Note:
This is an uncomplicated movement of massaging the ears to suit what makes you happy, soft and slow or hard and fast.
This is your time, enjoy.

Cool Down
3
Head flops

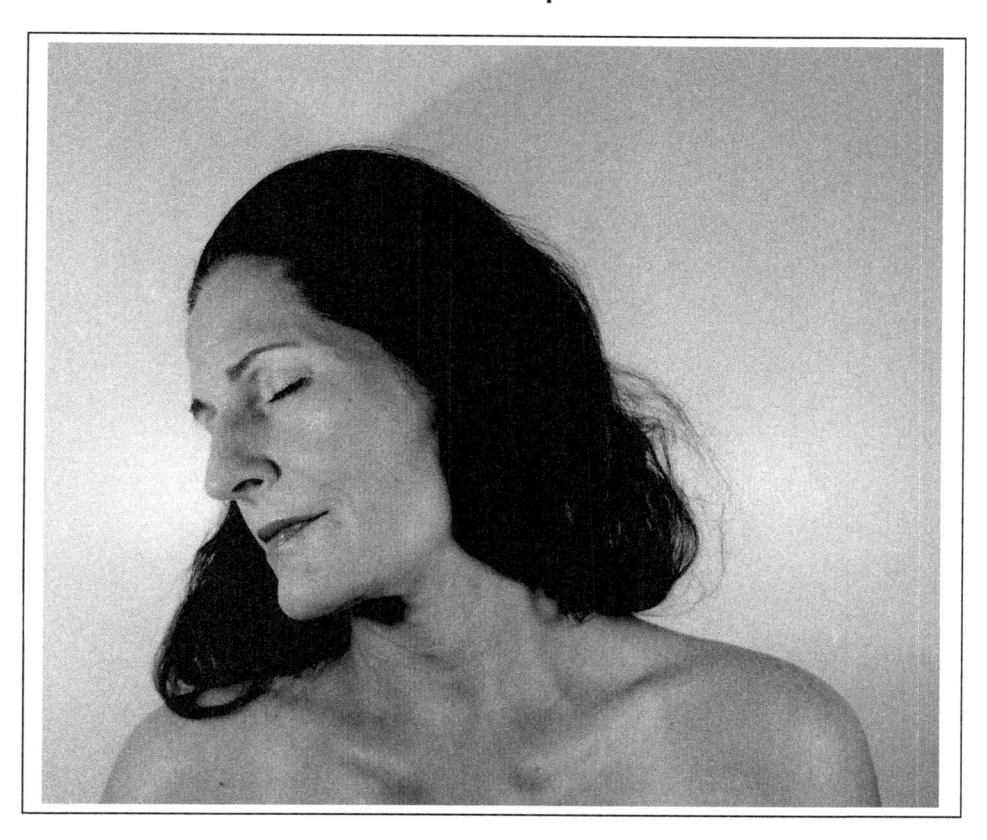

Keep shoulders back
Flop your head forwards, leave for 30 seconds and or lift a flopped head and move flopped head from side to side, flop, or circle, continue for your remaining time allocated

This is an uncomplicated movement of massaging the ears to suit what makes you happy, soft and slow or hard and fast.

Note:
This is your time, enjoy.

**Cool Down
4
Head claws**

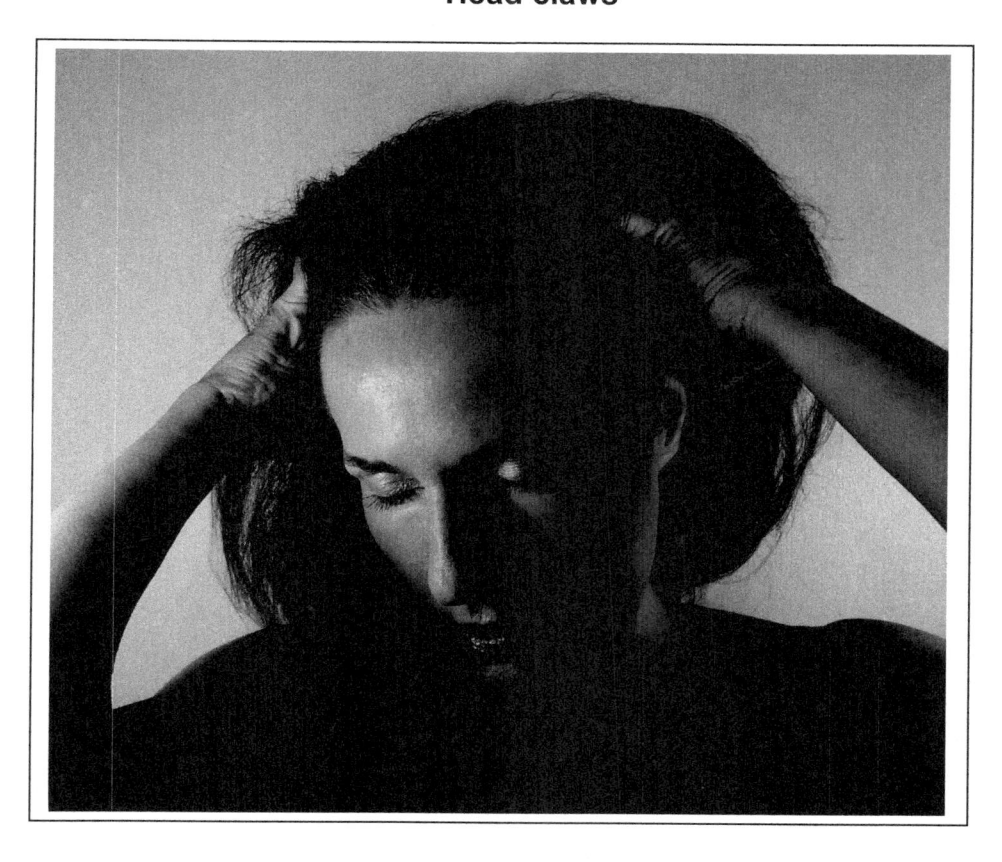

Place your hands on either side of head
Place your fingernails alongside the hairline of your scalp and draw fingernails through your hair to the crown of your head
Do it fast or slow, hard or softly - this is for you to enjoy

Repeat continuously for at least a minute

Note:
This is an uncomplicated movement of massaging the ears to suit what makes you happy, soft and slow or hard and fast.

This is your time, enjoy.